CLINICAL DECISION-MAKING IN DENTISTRY

Editor in Chief
Dr. Mattapudi Basavaiah Babu

Assistant Editor
Dr. Gauri Singh
Dr. Tanvi Saraf

NEXTGEN
SCHOLAR PUBLISHING

ISBN : 9788199862548

DOI : 10.5281/zenodo.18923410

Edition : First, March 2026

Title : Clinical Decision-Making in Dentistry

Editor : Dr. Mattapudi Basavaiah Babu, Dr. Gauri Singh, Dr. Tanvi Saraf

Published by

NEXTGEN SCHOLAR PUBLISHING

An Imprint of **Taneesha and Prachi NextGen Publication**

Registered Address: Plot No. 48, Road No. 2, Suman Nagar, Bahadarabad, Haridwar, Uttarakhand – 249402, India
Website : www.tpnextpub.com
E-mail : support@tpnextpub.com
Phone : +91 9760418103

Printed by :
Manipal Technologies Limited, Bengaluru - 560001, Karnataka

Index

Preface

Clinical dentistry today is no longer confined to the mechanical execution of procedures; it is an intellectual discipline rooted in analysis, interpretation, synthesis of evidence, and ethical responsibility. Every restoration placed, every extraction performed, every implant inserted, and every preventive strategy recommended is preceded—consciously or subconsciously—by a clinical decision. The quality of that decision ultimately determines the quality of care delivered.

In an era characterized by rapid technological advancements, expanding biomaterial innovations, digital workflows, artificial intelligence integration, and an ever-growing body of scientific literature, the contemporary dental practitioner faces a paradox of abundance: more choices, more data, more tools—yet greater complexity. Clinical Decision-Making in Dentistry is conceived to address this very challenge.

This book is founded on the principle that sound clinical judgment arises from the harmonious integration of three pillars:

1. Scientific evidence
2. Clinical expertise
3. Patient values and expectations

The framework echoes the philosophy of evidence-based healthcare pioneered by scholars such as David Sackett, yet contextualizes it within the unique biological, biomechanical, esthetic, and psychosocial dimensions of dentistry.

Modern dental decision-making demands more than diagnostic acumen; it requires awareness of cognitive biases, understanding of risk stratification, interdisciplinary coordination, prognostic foresight, ethical sensitivity, and cost–benefit reasoning. Whether deciding between endodontic retreatment and implant placement, selecting restorative biomaterials, planning phased periodontal therapy, or incorporating digital decision-support systems, clinicians must navigate uncertainty with structured reasoning.

This book has been systematically organized to mirror the real-world cognitive workflow of dental practice:

- Foundations of clinical reasoning and cognitive psychology
- Evidence integration and risk evaluation
- Diagnostic interpretation and treatment sequencing
- Specialty-specific decision pathways
- Management of complications and medico-legal considerations
- Ethical communication and shared decision-making
- Emerging digital and AI-driven tools for future practice

Each chapter emphasizes practical algorithms, risk-based thinking, and prognosis-driven planning while maintaining scientific rigor. The intent is not merely to present treatment modalities but to illuminate *why* and *when* specific interventions are appropriate.

Clinical decision-making is not static; it evolves with new evidence, technologies, and patient expectations. As artificial intelligence, machine learning, and predictive analytics increasingly enter dental diagnostics and treatment planning, the clinician's role transforms—from procedural operator to strategic healthcare decision architect.

This text is designed for postgraduate students, academicians, clinicians, and interdisciplinary specialists who seek to elevate their reasoning beyond protocol-driven practice toward thoughtful, individualized, evidence-informed care.

Ultimately, the objective of this book is simple yet profound: to cultivate clinicians who do not merely treat teeth—but who think critically, decide responsibly, and practice ethically.

Foundations of Clinical Decision-Making

Dr. Sugandha Sharma
MDS (Pediatric and Preventive Dentistry)
Consultant
Lather Dental Clinic and Implant Centre
Bhiwani

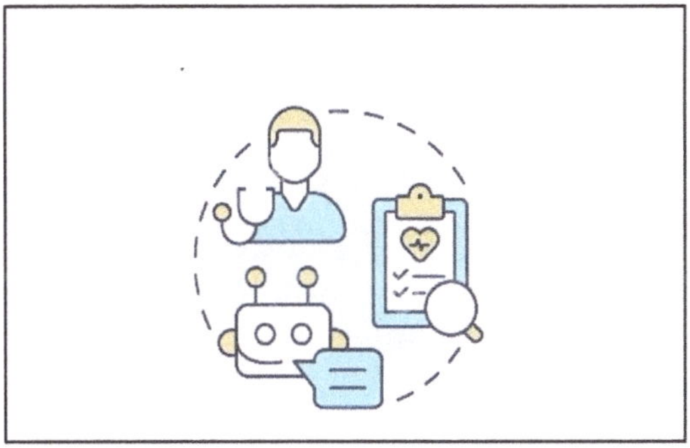

Introduction

Clinical dentistry is fundamentally a discipline of decision-making under uncertainty. Every patient encounter demands multiple layered judgments—diagnostic, prognostic, therapeutic, ethical, and economic. The clinician must interpret incomplete biological information, reconcile patient expectations with biological feasibility, evaluate evidence of variable quality, and predict long-term outcomes. Thus, clinical decision-making is not merely a technical adjunct to dental practice; it is its intellectual core. Historically, dental decisions were often guided by apprenticeship models, experiential learning, and authority-based teachings. However, modern dentistry operates in an evidence-rich, technologically advanced, and patient-centered environment. The evolution of evidence-based healthcare—formalized by pioneers such as David Sackett—shifted decision paradigms toward structured reasoning that integrates best evidence, clinical expertise, and patient values. Dentistry has since adapted these principles into evidence-based dentistry

(EBD), but the foundational cognitive architecture of decision-making warrants deeper exploration.

This chapter explores the conceptual foundations of clinical decision-making in dentistry, including its principles, theoretical models, cognitive psychology, and biases. It also provides structured frameworks and tables to facilitate systematic reasoning in everyday clinical practice.

1.1 The Nature of Clinical Decision-Making in Dentistry

Clinical decision-making can be defined as:

A systematic cognitive process through which a clinician gathers information, interprets findings, evaluates alternatives, predicts outcomes, and selects a course of action tailored to an individual patient.

Core Characteristics

1. Occurs under uncertainty
2. Is context-dependent
3. Is influenced by clinician experience
4. Involves probabilistic reasoning
5. Requires ethical justification
6. Must incorporate patient autonomy

Unlike algorithmic problem-solving in engineering, dental decision-making frequently deals with biological variability and patient-driven modifications. Two patients with identical radiographic lesions may require entirely different treatment plans based on risk factors, compliance, financial constraints, systemic health, and esthetic demands.

1.2 Principles of Sound Clinical Decision-Making

The foundation of rational decision-making rests on several guiding principles:

1. Patient-Centeredness

Treatment must align with patient values, cultural beliefs, systemic health, and socioeconomic considerations.

2. Evidence Integration

Clinical decisions should rely on current scientific literature, systematic reviews, and consensus guidelines.

3. Risk–Benefit Analysis

Each intervention must balance biological benefit against procedural risk.

4. Minimally Invasive Philosophy

Preservation of natural tissue remains paramount.

5. Prognosis-Oriented Planning

Every decision must consider long-term functional survival.

6. Ethical Accountability

The clinician must ensure transparency, informed consent, and fairness.

Table 1: Pillars of Clinical Decision-Making in Dentistry

Pillar	Description	Clinical Example
Biological	Disease severity, tissue condition	Caries depth assessment
Mechanical	Structural integrity, load distribution	Crown vs onlay decision
Patient-Centered	Expectations, affordability	Implant vs RPD
Evidence-Based	Literature support	Vital pulp therapy indications
Ethical	Consent, overtreatment avoidance	Avoiding unnecessary CBCT

1.3 Models of Clinical Decision-Making

Decision-making theories from medicine, psychology, and economics inform dental reasoning. These models can be broadly categorized into analytical and intuitive systems.

1.3.1 Hypothetico-Deductive Model

This classical clinical reasoning model involves:

1. Data collection

2. Hypothesis generation
3. Diagnostic testing
4. Hypothesis confirmation or rejection

In dentistry, this is commonly applied in endodontic diagnosis, where symptoms guide provisional hypotheses that are confirmed by pulp testing and radiographs.

1.3.2 Evidence-Based Decision Model

This triadic model integrates:

- Best available research evidence
- Clinical expertise
- Patient values

It formalizes decision-making and reduces reliance on anecdotal experience.

1.3.3 Dual-Process Theory

Derived from cognitive psychology, dual-process theory proposes two systems:

System	Characteristics	Dental Application
System 1	Fast, intuitive, pattern recognition	Immediate caries detection
System 2	Slow, analytical, deliberate	Complex implant planning

Experienced clinicians rely heavily on pattern recognition but must activate analytical reasoning in complex or unfamiliar cases.

1.3.4 Shared Decision-Making Model

Shared decision-making emphasizes collaborative planning between clinician and patient. It enhances compliance, trust, and ethical transparency.

Steps include:

1. Explain diagnosis

2. Present alternatives
3. Discuss risks and benefits
4. Explore patient preferences
5. Arrive at consensus

1.3.5 Decision Tree Analysis

Decision trees provide structured visualization of possible treatment pathways and outcomes, particularly useful in:

- Endodontic retreatment vs extraction
- Periodontal surgery vs maintenance
- Immediate vs delayed implant placement

Decision trees are structured, graphical representations of clinical reasoning that map out alternative treatment pathways, their possible consequences, and associated probabilities. They convert complex cognitive processes into visual logic sequences, making uncertainty explicit and outcomes measurable. In dentistry—where prognosis, risk factors, and patient preferences frequently intersect—decision trees enhance transparency, reduce bias, and support evidence-based choices.

Below is an elaborated explanation of how decision trees function in three common high-stakes dental scenarios, along with practical clinical examples.

1. Endodontic Retreatment vs Extraction

This is one of the most consequential decisions in restorative dentistry. The clinician must weigh biological feasibility, structural integrity, long-term survival, patient finances, and alternative replacement options.

Structure of the Decision Tree

Step 1: Initial Node (Decision Node)

Tooth with failed root canal treatment (symptomatic or persistent periapical lesion).

Two primary branches:

- Nonsurgical retreatment

- Extraction

Branch A: Endodontic Retreatment

Key Evaluation Criteria

- Restorability
- Remaining tooth structure
- Periodontal support
- Presence of vertical root fracture
- Quality of previous obturation
- Patient compliance

Possible Outcomes

- Successful healing
- Persistent infection
- Need for apical surgery
- Eventual extraction

Clinical Example

A 35-year-old patient presents with a previously treated mandibular first molar with persistent periapical radiolucency. The tooth has adequate ferrule, no periodontal pocketing, and no fracture lines visible radiographically.

Decision Tree Logic:

1. Is the tooth restorable? → Yes
2. Is there a vertical root fracture? → No
3. Adequate periodontal support? → Yes
4. Quality of previous obturation inadequate? → Yes

→ Retreatment recommended

Estimated success rate: 70–85% depending on case complexity. If healing occurs → Crown replacement and monitoring. If persistent lesion → Apical surgery or extraction.

Branch B: Extraction

Subsequent Sub-Branches

- No replacement

- Removable partial denture
- Fixed bridge
- Implant placement

Clinical Example

If the same tooth had:

- Extensive structural loss
- Subgingival caries below bone
- Deep isolated periodontal defect
- Suspected vertical root fracture

→ Extraction becomes more predictable.

The tree then expands:

Extraction →

Option 1: Implant (requires adequate bone volume)

Option 2: Fixed bridge (adjacent tooth preparation required)

Option 3: Removable prosthesis

Each branch includes cost, surgical risk, longevity, and maintenance considerations.

Why Decision Trees Help Here

- Prevents premature extraction due to commission bias
- Quantifies retreatment survival probabilities
- Encourages evaluation of long-term prosthetic burden
- Facilitates shared decision-making discussion

2. Periodontal Surgery vs Maintenance Therapy

Chronic periodontitis management often requires careful staging rather than immediate surgical intervention.

Initial Node

Patient with Stage III periodontitis after nonsurgical therapy.

Two main branches:

- Continue supportive periodontal therapy
- Surgical intervention

Branch A: Maintenance Therapy

Indications

- Pockets reduced to ≤5 mm
- Good plaque control
- No vertical defects requiring regeneration
- Stable attachment levels

Outcomes

- Disease stabilization
- Possible slow progression
- Need for later surgery

Clinical Example

A 50-year-old patient presents with 5 mm pockets post-scaling and root planing, no mobility, and excellent plaque control.

Decision Logic:

1. Are pockets >6 mm? → No
2. Is bleeding on probing persistent? → Minimal
3. Vertical defects present? → No

→ Continue maintenance at 3–4 month intervals.

Expected outcome: Stability with regular recall.

Branch B: Periodontal Surgery

Indications

- Persistent ≥6 mm pockets
- Vertical defects
- Furcation involvement
- Poor access for debridement

Sub-Branches

- Open flap debridement
- Regenerative surgery
- Resective surgery

Clinical Example

If the same patient had:

- 7 mm pockets
- Class II furcation
- Radiographic vertical defect

Decision Tree Logic:

1. Persistent deep pockets? → Yes
2. Regenerative potential? → Yes (vertical defect)
3. Patient compliant? → Yes

→ Regenerative surgery recommended.

Possible outcomes:

- Attachment gain
- Partial improvement
- Persistent defect

Why Decision Trees Help Here

- Avoids overtreatment
- Encourages staged therapy
- Integrates patient compliance into prognosis
- Aligns with minimally invasive philosophy

3. Immediate vs Delayed Implant Placement

Implant timing decisions depend on biological healing, infection control, bone availability, esthetics, and systemic health.

Initial Node

Non-restorable tooth indicated for extraction.

Two main branches:

- Immediate implant placement
- Delayed implant placement

Branch A: Immediate Implant

Indications

- Intact socket walls
- No acute infection
- Adequate apical bone

- Good systemic health
- Esthetic zone considerations

Advantages

- Reduced treatment time
- Fewer surgeries
- Preservation of soft tissue architecture

Risks

- Implant failure if infection persists
- Esthetic compromise if buccal plate thin

Clinical Example

A 28-year-old patient with fractured maxillary central incisor, intact buccal plate, no infection.

Decision Logic:

1. Active infection? → No
2. Adequate apical bone for primary stability? → Yes
3. Thin biotype? → Moderate

→ Immediate implant with provisionalization.

Expected survival: Comparable to delayed placement in ideal cases.

Branch B: Delayed Implant Placement

Indications

- Active infection
- Severe bone loss
- Buccal plate defect
- Systemic risk factors
- Poor oral hygiene

Sub-Branches

- Early placement (4–8 weeks)
- Late placement (3–6 months)
- Ridge preservation first

Clinical Example

A 60-year-old diabetic patient with abscessed mandibular molar and buccal plate loss.

Decision Logic:

1. Acute infection present? → Yes
2. Adequate bone for stability? → No
3. Systemic condition controlled? → Borderline

→ Extraction + ridge preservation → Delayed implant after healing.

Why Decision Trees Help Here

- Makes surgical timing explicit
- Integrates systemic health
- Reduces impulsive immediate placement
- Improves patient education

Structural Components of a Dental Decision Tree

A typical clinical decision tree includes:

1. Decision Node (square) – clinician choice
2. Chance Node (circle) – probability-based outcome
3. Outcome Node (triangle) – final result

Table: Key Variables Incorporated in Dental Decision Trees

Variable	Example
Biological status	Bone density, pulp vitality
Structural integrity	Remaining ferrule
Periodontal support	Attachment levels
Systemic health	Diabetes, smoking
Patient preference	Cost tolerance
Evidence-based prognosis	Survival rates

Clinical Advantages of Using Decision Trees

1. Enhances transparency in reasoning

2. Reduces cognitive bias
3. Facilitates documentation
4. Encourages risk-based thinking
5. Supports shared decision-making
6. Allows comparison of long-term survival probabilities

Limitations

- Requires reliable probability data
- Can oversimplify complex biological variables
- May not capture dynamic patient factors
- Time-consuming in busy practice

Table 2: Comparative Overview of Decision Models

Model	Strength	Limitation	Best Used In
Hypothetico-deductive	Structured reasoning	Time-consuming	Diagnosis
Dual-process	Efficient	Prone to bias	Routine practice
Evidence-based	Scientifically robust	Literature overload	Treatment selection
Shared decision-making	Ethical	Requires communication skill	Elective procedures
Decision tree	Visual clarity	Requires probability data	Prognosis evaluation

Integrated Decision Tree Tables in Dentistry

1. Endodontic Retreatment vs Extraction

Integrated Clinical Decision Tree Table

Step	Decision Node / Variable	Criteria Evaluated	If YES → Pathway	If NO → Pathway	Prognostic Consideration
1	Tooth previously root canal treated with persistent lesion	Clinical symptoms, radiographic lesion	Proceed to restorability assessment	Monitor if asymptomatic small lesion	Lesion size & duration influence healing
2	Is the tooth restorable?	Remaining ferrule, crown-root ratio, structural integrity	Evaluate for retreatment	Extraction indicated	Structural failure reduces long-term survival
3	Vertical root fracture present?	CBCT, isolated deep probing	Extraction	Continue evaluation	VRF → poor prognosis
4	Adequate periodontal support	Attachment level, mobility	Retreatment feasible	Extraction or periodontal therapy first	Combined endo-perio lowers

	?				survival
5	Cause of failure identifiable?	Missed canal, poor obturation	Nonsurgical retreatment	Consider apical surgery	Identifiable cause improves success (70–85%)
6	Retreatment successful?	6–12 month healing	Definitive restoration	Surgical intervention or extraction	Crown quality influences longevity
7	If extraction	Replacement decision	Implant / Bridge / RPD	No replacement	Implant survival ~90–95% (10 yrs)

Clinical Interpretation

This integrated model forces sequential biological validation before extraction. It reduces commission bias and ensures retreatment is considered when structural and periodontal parameters are favorable.

2. Periodontal Surgery vs Maintenance

Integrated Clinical Decision Tree Table

Step	Decisio	Assessmen	If	If	Progn

	n Node / Variable	**t Parameter**	**Favorable → Path**	**Unfavorable → Path**	**osis Impact**
1	Post-SRP evaluation (4–6 weeks)	Pocket depth measurement	≤5 mm → Maintenance	≥6 mm → Surgical evaluation	Residual depth predicts progression
2	Bleeding on probing	Inflammation control	Continue maintenance	Consider surgical therapy	Persistent bleeding indicates activity
3	Vertical bony defect present?	Radiograph, probing	Regenerative surgery	Open flap debridement	3-wall defects respond better
4	Furcation involvement	Glickman grade	Maintenance (Grade I)	Surgery (Grade II–III)	Furcation worsens prognosis
5	Patient compliance	Plaque index	Continue non-surgical	Surgery only if complia	Poor compliance

				nt	→ recurrence
6	Surgical outcome	Attachment gain	Maintenance phase	Re-evaluate or extraction	Maintenance critical for survival

Clinical Interpretation

This table ensures surgery is not first-line unless nonsurgical therapy fails. It integrates compliance as a decisive prognostic variable—often overlooked in intuitive decision-making.

3. Immediate vs Delayed Implant Placement

Integrated Clinical Decision Tree Table

Step	Decision Node / Variable	Clinical Assessment	Immediate Implant	Delayed Implant	Biological Rationale
1	Active infection present?	Abscess, suppuration	Avoid immediate	Extraction + healing	Infection compromises osseointegration
2	Intact socket walls?	Buccal plate integrity	Immediate feasible	Ridge preservation	Buccal plate loss →

					recession risk
3	Adequate apical bone for primary stability?	≥3–4 mm beyond apex	Immediate placement	Delayed placement	Primary stability critical
4	Soft tissue biotype	Thin vs thick	Consider grafting	Delayed may improve contour	Thin biotype ↑ recession risk
5	Systemic risk factors	Diabetes, smoking	Case-by-case	Prefer delayed	Healing capacity affects success
6	Esthetic zone?	Smile line, gingival display	Immediate provisional if ideal	Delayed with soft tissue conditioning	Esthetic predictability variable
7	Final outcome	Osseointegration success	Comparable survival in ideal cases	High predictability in compromised sites	Case selection determines success

Comparative Integrated Decision Overview

Clinical Scenario	Primary Biological Variable	Structural Variable	Patient Variable	Preferred Conservative Path
Failed RCT	Periapical pathology	Ferrule presence	Financial tolerance	Retreatment first
Periodontitis	Pocket depth	Bone defect morphology	Compliance	Maintenance before surgery
Implant timing	Infection status	Socket integrity	Systemic health	Immediate only if ideal

How to Use Integrated Decision Tables in Practice

1. Move sequentially from biological feasibility → structural assessment → patient-centered modifiers.

2. Avoid skipping steps (reduces anchoring bias).

3. Document each decision node in patient records.

4. Use tables during case discussions or interdisciplinary meetings.

5. Convert high-risk decisions into probability discussions with patients.

Advantages of Integrated Table-Based Decision Trees

- Converts abstract reasoning into structured logic
- Encourages prognosis-based sequencing
- Enhances medico-legal documentation
- Facilitates teaching for postgraduate programs
- Promotes minimally invasive philosophy
- Reduces cognitive bias

Conceptual Framework Summary

Decision-making in dentistry should proceed in the following hierarchical order:

Biological Possibility → Structural Feasibility → Periodontal Stability → Systemic Modifiers → Patient Preference → Long-Term Prognosis → Ethical Justification

1.4 Critical Thinking in Dentistry

Critical thinking is the disciplined intellectual process of actively analyzing, synthesizing, and evaluating information to guide action.

It involves:

- Logical reasoning
- Interpretation of diagnostic data
- Identification of assumptions
- Reflection on potential errors
- Evaluation of alternatives

In restorative dentistry, critical thinking is essential when deciding whether to repair or replace a restoration. The decision must evaluate marginal integrity, secondary caries risk, occlusal load, and patient caries risk profile.

Components of Critical Thinking

1. Interpretation
2. Analysis
3. Evaluation
4. Inference
5. Explanation
6. Self-regulation

Table 3: Critical Thinking Framework in Clinical Practice

Step	Clinical Question
Interpretation	What does the radiograph truly show?

Analysis	What are possible causes?
Evaluation	Which diagnosis is most probable?
Inference	What treatment logically follows?
Reflection	Could bias be influencing me?

1.5 Cognitive Biases in Dental Decision-Making

Cognitive biases are systematic errors in thinking that affect judgments. They are inherent to human cognition and influence both novice and experienced clinicians.

Understanding biases is crucial to minimizing diagnostic errors and overtreatment.

1.5.1 Common Cognitive Biases in Dentistry

1. Anchoring Bias

Relying heavily on initial information (e.g., first radiographic impression).

2. Confirmation Bias

Seeking information that supports an initial diagnosis.

3. Availability Bias

Overestimating conditions frequently encountered recently.

4. Overconfidence Bias

Overestimating personal skill or diagnostic accuracy.

5. Commission Bias

Preferring action over observation.

6. Framing Effect

Being influenced by how options are presented.

Cognitive biases are subtle yet powerful influences that shape clinical reasoning in everyday dental practice. They operate unconsciously, often emerging from pattern recognition, past experiences, time pressure, or emotional investment in a diagnosis. While experience enhances efficiency, it also increases vulnerability to systematic errors in judgment.

A deeper understanding of these biases allows the clinician to move from intuitive reaction to reflective, structured reasoning.

Anchoring bias occurs when a clinician fixates on the first piece of information obtained and allows it to disproportionately influence subsequent interpretation. Consider a patient presenting with mild discomfort and a periapical radiolucency associated with a previously restored mandibular molar. The radiographic image immediately suggests pulpal necrosis, and the clinician mentally commits to a diagnosis of chronic apical periodontitis. However, vitality testing is either skipped or superficially performed. In reality, the tooth may be vital, and the radiolucency could represent a non-endodontic lesion such as cemento-osseous dysplasia. The initial "anchor" — the radiograph — dominates the reasoning process, preventing a broader differential diagnosis. The result is misdiagnosis and potentially unnecessary root canal therapy. Anchoring is particularly common in high-volume practices where rapid visual impressions drive workflow efficiency.

Closely related is confirmation bias, wherein the clinician selectively seeks or interprets information that supports an initial assumption while discounting contradictory findings. For example, a patient complains of lingering cold sensitivity. The clinician suspects irreversible pulpitis and performs pulp testing. One test produces prolonged sensitivity, but percussion is negative, spontaneous pain is absent, and radiographs show no periapical changes. Instead of reconsidering the possibility of reversible pulpitis, the clinician emphasizes the lingering symptom as definitive evidence and proceeds with endodontic treatment. The desire to validate the preliminary diagnosis overrides balanced analysis. This bias can lead to overtreatment, especially in endodontics, where diagnostic thresholds are sometimes subjective.

Availability bias arises when recent or memorable clinical experiences disproportionately influence diagnostic probability. Suppose a clinician has recently treated several patients with temporomandibular disorders (TMD). Shortly thereafter, a new patient presents with unilateral facial pain radiating toward the ear. Because TMD cases are fresh in memory, the clinician quickly attributes the symptoms to myofascial pain dysfunction without conducting a comprehensive pulpal, periodontal, and sinus evaluation. The actual cause may be symptomatic irreversible pulpitis in a maxillary molar or even maxillary sinusitis. The ease with which TMD comes to mind inflates its perceived likelihood. Availability bias tends to increase after exposure to unusual or emotionally charged cases, subtly distorting diagnostic calibration.

Overconfidence bias reflects an inflated belief in one's diagnostic accuracy or procedural competence. This bias often develops with increasing clinical experience. For instance, during endodontic retreatment of a mandibular molar, the clinician elects not to obtain a CBCT scan, confident in their ability to locate all canals based on prior experience. However, a missed middle mesial canal results in persistent infection and eventual failure. Overconfidence may reduce the perceived need for adjunctive imaging, specialist referral, or second opinions. While confidence is essential for decisive care, excessive confidence reduces diagnostic vigilance and increases complication risk.

Commission bias describes the tendency to favor action over inaction, even when observation may be the more appropriate course. A borderline tooth with moderate periodontal bone loss, questionable crown-to-root ratio, and manageable mobility presents a prognostic dilemma. Rather than implementing periodontal stabilization and monitoring, the clinician recommends extraction and implant placement, believing that active intervention equates to better care. In some cases, conservative management could have preserved the natural tooth for years. Commission bias is reinforced by procedural training environments, patient expectations for definitive solutions, and financial incentives tied to operative interventions. The risk is overtreatment and loss of biologically salvageable structures.

These cognitive biases rarely occur in isolation. Anchoring may initiate a diagnostic pathway, confirmation bias may reinforce it, availability bias may distort probability assessment, overconfidence may reduce verification, and commission bias may accelerate intervention. The cumulative effect can compromise biological outcomes and ethical integrity. Recognizing these biases requires deliberate reflective practice. Structured diagnostic checklists, systematic vitality testing protocols, peer discussion, and activation of slow analytical reasoning can interrupt intuitive errors. In complex or high-risk decisions, consciously asking, "What else could this be?" or "What evidence contradicts my assumption?" can recalibrate judgment.

Ultimately, expertise in dentistry is not the absence of bias but the awareness of it. Clinical maturity lies in balancing intuition with analysis, speed with reflection, and confidence with humility. By acknowledging and mitigating cognitive biases, clinicians elevate decision-making from habitual pattern recognition to disciplined, patient-centered reasoning.

Table 4: Cognitive Biases and Clinical Examples

Bias	Clinical Example	Risk
Anchoring	Assuming periapical lesion is endodontic without vitality testing	Misdiagnosis
Confirmation	Ignoring contradictory pulp test	Inappropriate RCT
Availability	Diagnosing TMD due to recent similar cases	Overdiagnosis
Overconfidence	Skipping CBCT for complex canal	Missed anatomy
Commission	Extracting borderline tooth instead of monitoring	Overtreatment

1.6 Strategies to Minimize Cognitive Bias

1. Structured diagnostic checklists
2. Second opinions
3. Reflective practice
4. Evidence consultation
5. Multidisciplinary discussion
6. Use of decision-support tools

Cognitive bias in dentistry cannot be eliminated, for it is intrinsic to human cognition; however, it can be systematically attenuated through deliberate intellectual discipline and structured safeguards embedded within clinical workflow. The first and perhaps most practical strategy involves the implementation of structured diagnostic checklists. Checklists function as cognitive forcing tools—they compel the clinician to verify essential parameters before committing to a diagnosis or treatment plan. In endodontics, for example, a checklist requiring vitality testing, percussion, palpation, periodontal probing, radiographic interpretation, and differential diagnosis documentation prevents premature anchoring on a single radiographic finding. By externalizing the reasoning process, checklists reduce reliance on intuitive pattern recognition alone and minimize omission errors that arise from time pressure or cognitive overload.

Equally critical is the cultivation of second opinions, whether through peer consultation, specialist referral, or interdisciplinary case review. A second opinion introduces an independent cognitive framework that may identify blind spots or challenge untested assumptions. In implant planning, for instance, a prosthodontist may detect restorative limitations that a surgically focused clinician might overlook. The act of inviting external scrutiny not only mitigates overconfidence bias but also strengthens medico-legal defensibility by demonstrating due diligence in complex cases. Reflective practice represents a more internal yet profoundly transformative strategy. It requires clinicians to consciously revisit their diagnostic reasoning, particularly in cases of unexpected outcomes or complications. Reflection transforms experience into calibrated expertise. By asking, "What assumptions did I make?" or "Was there evidence I ignored?" the practitioner develops metacognitive awareness—the capacity to think about one's own thinking. Over time, reflective documentation in clinical notes enhances self-regulation and reduces repetitive cognitive errors.

Evidence consultation further anchors decision-making in scientifically validated data rather than anecdotal memory. Consulting systematic reviews, consensus guidelines, and contemporary clinical trials counteracts availability bias, which tends to overemphasize recent or memorable cases. For example, reviewing survival data before recommending extraction versus retreatment ensures that the decision reflects population-level outcomes rather than isolated personal experiences. Evidence-based consultation recalibrates subjective probability into objective risk estimation.

Multidisciplinary discussion expands this corrective mechanism by integrating diverse professional perspectives. Periodontal, endodontic, prosthodontic, and surgical viewpoints often illuminate variables that a single-discipline lens may neglect. Complex cases involving compromised teeth, occlusal instability, or esthetic demands benefit from collaborative reasoning. Multidisciplinary dialogue dilutes individual cognitive bias by distributing responsibility across a collective analytical process, thereby enhancing biological predictability and ethical transparency.

Finally, the integration of decision-support tools—including digital diagnostic software, risk assessment algorithms, and artificial intelligence–based imaging analysis—provides an additional structural safeguard. These tools, when used judiciously, serve as adjunctive analytical systems that complement clinical intuition. For instance, caries risk assessment models standardize evaluation criteria, while CBCT software assists in identifying anatomical complexities that may be overlooked visually. However, technological assistance must itself be critically appraised to avoid automation bias; the clinician must remain the ultimate arbiter of judgment. In synthesis, minimizing cognitive bias requires a multilayered defense: structured protocols to prevent omission, collaborative consultation to challenge assumptions, reflective introspection to refine reasoning, evidence alignment to recalibrate probabilities, interdisciplinary discourse to broaden perspective, and technological augmentation to enhance diagnostic precision. When these strategies are integrated into routine practice, clinical decision-making evolves from intuitive habit to disciplined intellectual craftsmanship, thereby elevating both patient safety and professional integrity.

Table 5: Bias Mitigation Framework

Strategy	Mechanism	Application
Diagnostic checklist	Reduces omission errors	Endodontic diagnosis
Peer review	External perspective	Implant planning
Slow thinking activation	Engages analytical reasoning	Complex prosthodontics
Literature consultation	Evidence correction	Material selection

1.7 Clinical Uncertainty and Probabilistic Thinking

Dentistry operates on probabilities rather than certainties. Prognosis must be estimated using risk assessment models, survival studies, and clinician experience.

For example:

- A cracked tooth may have uncertain pulpal prognosis
- Periodontal prognosis depends on patient compliance
- Implant survival varies with systemic risk factors

Clinicians must communicate uncertainty transparently.

Dentistry, unlike the deterministic sciences, functions within a probabilistic biological environment where outcomes are influenced by host response, microbial variability, mechanical loading, systemic health, and patient behavior. Absolute certainty is rarely attainable; rather, clinicians estimate prognosis through a synthesis of risk assessment models, longitudinal survival studies, and calibrated clinical experience. A cracked tooth, for instance, may present with minimal symptoms and normal vitality testing, yet the pulpal prognosis remains guarded because microfracture propagation and bacterial ingress cannot be predicted with precision.

Similarly, periodontal stability is not determined solely by initial attachment levels but is profoundly influenced by patient compliance with plaque control and maintenance visits; identical clinical parameters may yield divergent long-term outcomes depending on behavioral adherence. Implant survival, often reported with high cumulative success rates, is nevertheless modulated by systemic risk factors such as uncontrolled diabetes, smoking, osteoporosis, or parafunctional habits, each altering osseointegration dynamics and peri-implant tissue stability. In this landscape of biological variability, transparent communication of uncertainty becomes both an ethical and medico-legal imperative.

The clinician must articulate that treatment recommendations are based on current evidence and probability—not guarantees—while documenting the discussion of risks, alternatives, and potential complications. For example, if a cracked tooth is treated conservatively with full-coverage restoration and later progresses to pulpal necrosis requiring endodontic therapy, prior documentation that the pulpal prognosis was "guarded" and that the patient was informed of possible future root canal treatment provides critical medico-legal protection. Courts and regulatory bodies do not expect infallibility; they expect reasonable, evidence-based judgment and informed consent. Thus, acknowledging uncertainty does not weaken professional authority; rather, it strengthens ethical integrity, fosters patient trust, and safeguards against allegations of negligence arising from biologically unpredictable outcomes.

1.8 Ethical Dimensions of Decision-Making

Ethical decision-making is inseparable from clinical reasoning. Core principles include:

1. Autonomy
2. Beneficence
3. Non-maleficence
4. Justice

Overtreatment, unnecessary radiographs, or material upselling violate ethical integrity.

Table 6: Ethical Conflicts in Dental Decisions

Scenario	Ethical Concern	Resolution
Replacing functioning amalgam for esthetics	Beneficence vs commercial gain	Shared decision
Implant in poorly controlled diabetic	Risk vs autonomy	Medical clearance
CBCT for simple extraction	Radiation exposure	ALARA principle

1.9 Integration of Clinical Judgment

True expertise arises from calibrated experience. With increasing clinical exposure, pattern recognition improves; however, vigilance against bias must also increase.

Expert clinicians:

- Recognize limits of knowledge
- Seek evidence updates
- Balance intuition with analysis

- Communicate transparently
- Document rationale clearly

1.10 Future Perspective of Foundational Decision-Making

The emergence of artificial intelligence, predictive analytics, and digital diagnostic algorithms will not replace clinicians but augment structured reasoning. However, reliance on technology without foundational cognitive discipline risks automation bias.

Thus, mastering foundational principles remains indispensable before embracing advanced tools.

Evidence-Based Dentistry

Dr. Deepshikha Rodricks
Senior lecturer
Department of Oral Medicine and Radiology
Late Shri Yashwantrao Chavan Memorial Medical & Rural Development Foundation's Dental College & Hospital, Ahilyanagar
Maharashtra

Integrating clinical expertise, patient values, and best available evidence.

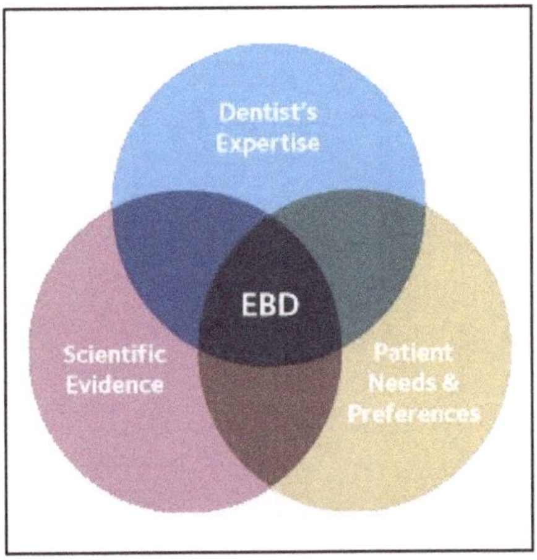

Evidence-Based Dentistry (EBD) represents a paradigm shift from authority-driven or tradition-based practice toward structured, transparent, and scientifically grounded clinical reasoning. It is not merely the application of research findings to patient care; rather, it is the conscientious integration of three interdependent pillars: best available scientific evidence, clinician expertise, and patient values and circumstances. When harmonized, these components create a calibrated framework for rational, ethical, and patient-centered decision-making.

The conceptual roots of evidence-based practice are traced to the evidence-based medicine movement articulated by David Sackett, who defined it as the integration of best research evidence with clinical expertise and patient values. Dentistry subsequently adapted this philosophy to its unique biological and biomechanical complexities. In modern dental care—where biomaterials evolve rapidly, digital diagnostics proliferate, and patient expectations intensify—the disciplined application of evidence is no longer optional but foundational.

The Three Pillars of Evidence-Based Dentistry

EBD rests upon a triadic structure, each component indispensable and mutually reinforcing.

1. Best Available Scientific Evidence

This includes systematically appraised research, such as randomized controlled trials (RCTs), cohort studies, systematic reviews, and meta-analyses. Scientific evidence informs probability estimates, comparative effectiveness, and long-term survival outcomes.

However, not all evidence is equal. The hierarchy of evidence places systematic reviews and meta-analyses at the apex, followed by RCTs, observational studies, and expert opinion. Yet hierarchy alone does not determine applicability. External validity—whether study findings are generalizable to the individual patient—remains critical.

2. Clinical Expertise

Clinical expertise encompasses the practitioner's accumulated experience, diagnostic acumen, technical skills, and judgment developed through reflective practice. Expertise enables contextual interpretation of evidence. A systematic review may report comparable survival rates for two restorative materials, but the clinician must evaluate handling properties, esthetic demands, occlusal load, and patient compliance before selecting one.

3. Patient Values and Preferences

Patients bring unique cultural, financial, psychological, and functional considerations. A technically ideal treatment may be unacceptable to a patient due to cost, invasiveness, or time commitment. True evidence-based care requires shared decision-making in which patient autonomy shapes final treatment selection.

Table 1: The Core Triad of Evidence-Based Dentistry

Component	Description	Clinical Example
Best Evidence	Scientifically validated research	Survival data comparing implants vs bridges
Clinical Expertise	Skill and experiential judgment	Assessing ferrule effect before crown placement
Patient Values	Preferences, affordability, expectations	Choosing removable prosthesis over implant due to cost

The EBD Process: Structured Application

Evidence-based dentistry is not theoretical; it follows a systematic methodology.

1. Formulate a focused clinical question
2. Search for relevant evidence
3. Critically appraise the evidence
4. Apply findings in context
5. Evaluate outcomes

The PICO framework (Population, Intervention, Comparison, Outcome) is commonly used to structure clinical questions.

Table 2: Example of PICO Application in Dentistry

Component	Example Scenario
Population	Adults with failed root canal treatment
Intervention	Nonsurgical retreatment
Comparison	Extraction and implant placement
Outcome	Long-term survival and complication rate

Using PICO clarifies the clinical dilemma and directs literature search toward focused evidence rather than anecdotal data.

Clinical Application: A Narrative Example

Consider a 40-year-old patient presenting with a previously treated maxillary molar exhibiting persistent periapical radiolucency. The clinician must decide between endodontic retreatment and extraction followed by implant placement.

Best Evidence:

Systematic reviews suggest that well-executed nonsurgical retreatment may achieve survival rates comparable to implants over medium-term follow-up in restorable teeth.

Clinical Expertise:

The clinician evaluates remaining tooth structure, crown margin integrity, periodontal support, and occlusal scheme. The presence of adequate ferrule and absence of vertical root fracture improve prognosis.

Patient Values:

The patient expresses concern about surgical intervention and higher implant costs but desires long-term stability.

After integrating these three domains, retreatment becomes the preferred first-line option. If biological or structural limitations had been present, extraction might have been more appropriate. The decision, therefore, is not dictated solely by literature nor solely by operator preference, but by structured integration.

Critical Appraisal and Interpretation of Evidence

Merely accessing research is insufficient; clinicians must evaluate:

- Study design
- Sample size
- Follow-up duration
- Risk of bias
- Statistical significance vs clinical relevance

For instance, a statistically significant difference between two restorative materials may not translate into clinically meaningful longevity differences. Similarly, short-term survival studies cannot reliably predict 10-year outcomes.

Table 3: Appraisal Criteria for Dental Research

Criterion	Clinical Significance
Randomization	Reduces selection bias
Blinding	Minimizes observer bias
Adequate follow-up	Ensures validity of survival data
Confidence intervals	Indicates precision of estimate
Applicability	Determines real-world relevance

Challenges in Evidence-Based Dentistry

Despite its strengths, EBD faces practical limitations:

1. Limited high-quality RCTs in certain dental domains
2. Rapid technological evolution outpacing long-term data
3. Industry-sponsored studies introducing bias
4. Variability in operator skill affecting reproducibility
5. Time constraints in busy clinical settings

Moreover, dentistry frequently deals with procedural interventions that are difficult to blind or standardize across operators, making absolute evidence synthesis complex.

Integrating Risk Assessment Models

Modern EBD increasingly incorporates risk-based frameworks. Caries risk assessment, periodontal staging and grading, and implant risk stratification models enhance individualized prediction. Evidence provides general probabilities; risk models personalize them.

For example:

- A smoker's implant survival probability differs from that of a non-smoker.
- High caries risk patients may benefit from minimally invasive restorations supported by preventive protocols.

Thus, evidence must be contextualized within individualized risk profiles.

Shared Decision-Making and Ethical Transparency

Evidence without communication fails its ethical purpose. Shared decision-making requires:

1. Explanation of diagnosis
2. Discussion of alternatives
3. Presentation of risks and benefits
4. Clarification of uncertainties
5. Documentation of consent

Patients must understand that recommendations are probability-based, not guarantees. Transparent communication strengthens trust and therapeutic alliance.

Table 4: Integrating Evidence with Patient Communication

Clinical Situation	Evidence Input	Patient Discussion Focus
Implant placement	10-year survival data	Surgical risk, maintenance needs
Vital pulp therapy	Success rates in mature teeth	Possibility of later RCT
Periodontal surgery	Attachment gain averages	Compliance requirement

Ethical and Medico-Legal Implications

Evidence-based dentistry carries profound medico-legal significance. Courts and regulatory authorities increasingly evaluate whether a clinician's decision aligns with accepted scientific standards rather than personal opinion. Failure to consult current guidelines or to inform patients of evidence-supported alternatives may constitute negligence.

For example, if a clinician extracts a restorable tooth without discussing retreatment options supported by survival data, and the patient later claims unnecessary extraction, documented evidence consultation and discussion of alternatives become critical defensive elements. Conversely, recommending an implant in a medically compromised patient without disclosing increased failure risk may expose the practitioner to allegations of inadequate informed consent.

Documentation should reflect:

- Evidence considered
- Alternatives discussed
- Risks explained
- Patient's informed preference

Evidence-based reasoning thus provides both biological justification and medico-legal protection. It demonstrates that decisions were not arbitrary but grounded in scientific rationale and ethical transparency.

Patient Assessment and Risk Evaluation

Dr. Samra Shafique
Senior lecturer
Department of conservative dentistry and endodontics
Sardar Patel post graduate institute of dental and medical sciences
Lucknow

Medical history, dental history, caries risk, periodontal risk, and systemic considerations.

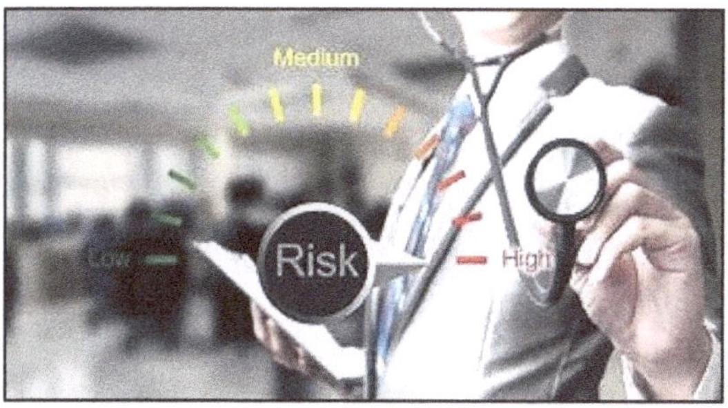

Patient assessment is the intellectual and biological cornerstone of clinical decision-making in dentistry. Before a bur touches enamel or a surgical flap is reflected, the clinician must construct a comprehensive risk profile that integrates systemic health, oral disease history, behavioral patterns, environmental exposures, and psychosocial determinants. Treatment without structured assessment is procedural; treatment grounded in risk evaluation is strategic.

Modern dentistry has transitioned from a lesion-based model to a risk-based paradigm. Rather than merely diagnosing existing pathology, clinicians are increasingly tasked with predicting disease susceptibility, estimating progression rates, and individualizing preventive and therapeutic strategies. This predictive approach enhances long-term stability, minimizes overtreatment, and aligns with ethical, patient-centered care. Patient assessment in dentistry can be conceptualized as a multilayered framework:

1. Medical history evaluation
2. Dental history assessment
3. Caries risk evaluation
4. Periodontal risk profiling
5. Systemic-dental interrelationships
6. Behavioral and lifestyle modifiers
7. Prognostic synthesis and documentation

- Each component interacts dynamically with the others, forming a biologically integrated clinical portrait.

1. Medical History Assessment

A thorough medical history is not a formality; it is a predictive tool. Many dental complications arise not from local pathology but from systemic interactions. The clinician must evaluate diseases, medications, allergies, hospitalizations, surgical history, and family predispositions.

1.1 Cardiovascular Disorders

Patients with hypertension, ischemic heart disease, arrhythmias, or prior myocardial infarction require careful stress management and pharmacologic considerations.

Example:

A 65-year-old patient with controlled hypertension on beta-blockers presents for multiple extractions. Vasoconstrictor-containing local anesthetics must be used cautiously, with aspiration and minimal effective dosage. Blood pressure should be recorded before treatment. Excessive epinephrine may precipitate tachyarrhythmia.

In patients with recent myocardial infarction (within 6 months), elective dental treatment should generally be deferred unless medically cleared.

1.2 Diabetes Mellitus

Diabetes significantly influences periodontal healing, infection susceptibility, implant survival, and wound repair.

Example:

A patient with poorly controlled diabetes (HbA1c >8%) presents for implant placement. Delayed osseointegration and increased peri-implantitis risk must be discussed. Glycemic stabilization prior to surgical intervention enhances prognosis.

Conversely, a well-controlled diabetic patient may demonstrate implant survival comparable to non-diabetics, illustrating the importance of metabolic control in risk stratification.

1.3 Bleeding Disorders and Anticoagulation

Patients on anticoagulants require coordinated management.

Example:

A patient taking warfarin with INR of 2.5 presents for surgical extraction. Minor oral surgery can typically proceed with local hemostatic measures if INR is within therapeutic range. Discontinuation of anticoagulant without physician consultation may increase thromboembolic risk.

1.4 Immunocompromised States

Patients undergoing chemotherapy, radiation therapy, or immunosuppressive therapy have altered healing capacity.

Patients treated with antiresorptive drugs (e.g., bisphosphonates) have risk of medication-related osteonecrosis of the jaw (MRONJ). Surgical decisions must consider duration and route of therapy.

1.5 Respiratory Conditions

Asthma and chronic obstructive pulmonary disease may influence positioning, sedation decisions, and material selection (avoid sulfite-containing anesthetics in sensitive individuals).

1.6 Pregnancy

Elective procedures are ideally deferred to the second trimester. Radiographs should be minimized and taken with shielding. Periodontal inflammation may be exacerbated by hormonal changes.

Table 1: Systemic Conditions and Dental Modifications

Systemic Condition	Dental	Risk Impact

	Consideration	
Diabetes	Delayed healing, implant caution	Increased infection risk
Hypertension	Stress reduction, epinephrine limitation	Cardiovascular events
Anticoagulation	Hemostasis management	Bleeding
Osteoporosis (bisphosphonate use)	Avoid elective surgery	MRONJ
Immunosuppression	Prophylaxis, healing monitoring	Post-op complications

2. Dental History Assessment

Past dental experiences shape biological and psychological outcomes. A detailed dental history reveals patterns of disease progression, compliance, and restorative longevity.

2.1 Previous Caries Experience

Caries is a disease of recurrence. Past caries activity is one of the strongest predictors of future lesions.

Example:

A 22-year-old with multiple restorations placed in the past three years likely represents high caries risk, even if current oral hygiene appears acceptable.

2.2 Endodontic History

Repeated root canal treatments may suggest structural compromise, occlusal overload, or recurrent caries.

2.3 Periodontal History

History of periodontal therapy, surgical intervention, and maintenance frequency strongly predicts stability.

Example:

A patient with prior periodontal surgery but irregular maintenance visits presents with recurrent attachment loss. Noncompliance modifies prognosis more than surgical technique.

2.4 Prosthodontic and Implant History

Repeated crown failure or implant complications may indicate occlusal discrepancies or parafunctional habits.

3. Caries Risk Assessment

Caries is a multifactorial biofilm-mediated disease influenced by microbial load, diet, saliva, fluoride exposure, and host factors.

Modern caries management emphasizes risk-based preventive strategies rather than purely restorative intervention.

3.1 Risk Factors

- High sugar intake frequency
- Reduced salivary flow
- Poor oral hygiene
- Orthodontic appliances
- Low fluoride exposure
- Socioeconomic factors

3.2 Clinical Indicators

- Active white spot lesions
- Multiple restorations
- Recurrent caries
- Visible plaque accumulation

Table 2: Caries Risk Stratification

Risk Level	Indicators	Management Strategy
Low	No new lesions in 3	Routine recall

	years	
Moderate	Occasional lesions	Fluoride varnish, diet counseling
High	Multiple new lesions, xerostomia	3-month recall, remineralization therapy

3.3 Clinical Example

A 45-year-old xerostomic patient on antidepressants presents with cervical lesions and rampant caries. Salivary flow testing confirms hyposalivation. Risk-based management includes prescription fluoride toothpaste, salivary substitutes, dietary modification, and shortened recall intervals. Restorative treatment alone would fail without addressing underlying risk.

4. Periodontal Risk Evaluation

Periodontal disease progression depends on host response, microbial challenge, systemic factors, and behavioral compliance.

4.1 Risk Indicators

- Smoking
- Diabetes
- Poor plaque control
- Genetic predisposition
- History of attachment loss

4.2 Staging and Grading

Modern classification emphasizes stage (severity) and grade (progression risk).

Example:

Stage III Grade C periodontitis in a smoker indicates high progression risk and requires aggressive intervention and strict maintenance.

Table 3: Periodontal Risk Factors and Impact

Factor	Effect on Disease	Prognostic Influence
Smoking	Impaired healing	Increased recurrence
Diabetes	Exaggerated inflammation	Rapid progression
Poor compliance	Plaque accumulation	Attachment loss
Genetic factors	Host susceptibility	Variable response

5. Systemic-Oral Interrelationships

Oral health and systemic health are bidirectionally linked.

5.1 Diabetes and Periodontitis

Chronic hyperglycemia exacerbates inflammatory cytokine release, increasing periodontal destruction. Conversely, periodontal therapy may modestly improve glycemic control.

5.2 Cardiovascular Disease

Periodontal pathogens have been implicated in systemic inflammation and endothelial dysfunction.

5.3 Osteoporosis

Reduced bone mineral density may influence alveolar bone stability and implant planning.

6. Behavioral and Lifestyle Factors

- Tobacco use
- Alcohol consumption
- Diet patterns
- Stress

• Parafunctional habits (bruxism)

Bruxism may compromise implant survival and fracture ceramic restorations.

7. Integrative Risk Synthesis

Comprehensive risk evaluation synthesizes all variables into an individualized prognosis.

Table 4: Comprehensive Risk Integration Matrix

Domain	Low Risk	Moderate Risk	High Risk
Medical	Healthy	Controlled systemic disease	Uncontrolled systemic disease
Caries	No recent lesions	Occasional lesions	Multiple active lesions
Periodontal	Stable	Mild attachment loss	Advanced periodontitis
Behavioral	Good compliance	Irregular hygiene	Smoking, poor hygiene

8. Clinical Case Integration

Case Example:

A 58-year-old smoker with controlled diabetes presents with moderate periodontitis and missing mandibular molars requesting implants.

Risk considerations:

• Smoking → Increased peri-implantitis risk

• Diabetes → Healing modulation

• Periodontal history → Recurrence potential

Management:

• Smoking cessation counselling

- Periodontal stabilization
- Glycemic monitoring
- Delayed implant placement with strict maintenance

9. Documentation and Medico-Legal Implications

Risk assessment documentation is a critical medico-legal safeguard. Courts evaluate whether the clinician:

- Identified systemic risk factors
- Communicated potential complications
- Offered alternatives
- Documented informed consent

If a diabetic smoker develops peri-implantitis after implant placement, documented evidence that increased risk was explained and discussed significantly strengthens legal defense.

Failure to assess medical history adequately—such as performing surgical extraction without identifying anticoagulant therapy—may constitute negligence.

Diagnostic Tools and Imaging

Dr. Madhu Arora
MDS, Reader
department of oral medicine and radiology
ITS dental college and hospital greater Noida

Clinical examination, radiography, CBCT, adjunctive diagnostic aids, and interpretation.

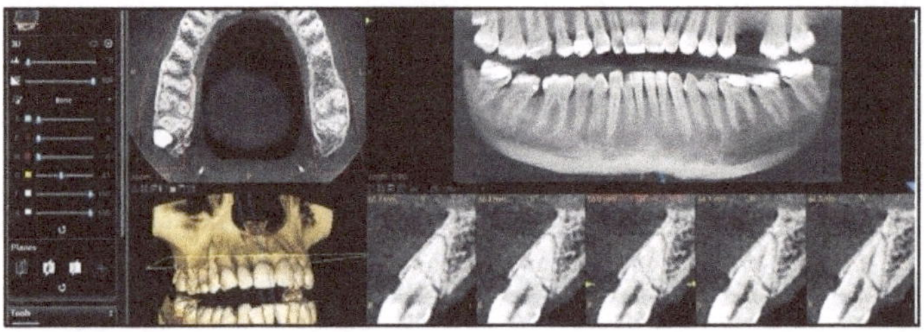

Accurate diagnosis forms the intellectual foundation of all dental treatment. Before restorative, endodontic, periodontal, prosthodontic, or surgical interventions are considered, the clinician must establish a precise understanding of disease presence, extent, severity, and prognosis. Diagnostic tools and imaging modalities transform subjective symptoms into objective data, enabling rational treatment planning grounded in evidence and clinical judgment. Modern dentistry integrates traditional clinical examination with advanced imaging technologies such as cone-beam computed tomography (CBCT), digital radiography, optical diagnostics, and adjunctive biomarker testing. Yet no single diagnostic method is definitive in isolation. Interpretation requires synthesis of patient history, clinical findings, imaging results, and risk assessment within a probability-based framework.

This narrative explores diagnostic tools in dentistry from an academic perspective, examining methodology, indications, interpretation principles, limitations, and clinical examples across disciplines.

I. Clinical Examination

Clinical examination remains the primary and indispensable diagnostic tool. Imaging and technology supplement—but never replace—structured clinical assessment.

1. Extraoral Examination

The extraoral examination evaluates:

- Facial symmetry
- Swellings or asymmetry
- Temporomandibular joint (TMJ) function
- Lymphadenopathy
- Skin lesions
- Muscular tenderness

For example, unilateral facial swelling associated with tenderness and fever may suggest acute odontogenic infection. In contrast, a firm, non-tender swelling with gradual enlargement may indicate a benign neoplasm.

TMJ examination includes palpation, range of motion measurement, deviation on opening, and auscultation for clicking or crepitus. Limited opening with deviation toward one side may suggest internal derangement.

2. Intraoral Soft Tissue Examination

Systematic soft tissue evaluation includes:

- Labial and buccal mucosa
- Gingiva
- Tongue (dorsal, ventral, lateral borders)
- Floor of mouth
- Hard and soft palate
- Oropharynx

Lesions are described using standardized criteria:

- Size
- Shape
- Color
- Surface texture

- Borders
- Consistency
- Duration

For instance, a non-healing ulcer on the lateral border of the tongue persisting beyond two weeks warrants further investigation and possible biopsy.

3. Hard Tissue Examination

The dental hard tissue examination evaluates:

- Caries presence
- Fractures
- Attrition/abrasion/erosion
- Existing restorations
- Occlusion

Visual-tactile inspection remains fundamental. Use of adequate illumination, magnification, and drying enhances detection.

Example:

A chalky white lesion near the gingival margin may indicate early enamel demineralization (incipient caries), whereas a cavitated brown lesion represents established decay.

4. Periodontal Examination

Periodontal assessment includes:

- Probing depth
- Clinical attachment level
- Bleeding on probing
- Furcation involvement
- Tooth mobility
- Plaque index

A 6 mm probing depth with bleeding suggests active periodontal inflammation. Radiographic correlation determines bone loss pattern.

5. Pulp Vitality Testing

Diagnostic methods include:

- Thermal testing (cold/hot)
- Electric pulp testing
- Percussion
- Palpation

Interpretation must be cautious. A delayed lingering response to cold often indicates irreversible pulpitis, whereas no response may suggest necrosis.

II. Radiography in Dentistry

Radiography translates anatomical and pathological changes into two-dimensional representations. Despite technological advances, conventional radiographs remain central in diagnosis.

Principles of Dental Radiography

- X-rays pass through tissues at varying absorption rates
- Dense structures appear radiopaque
- Less dense areas appear radiolucent
- Interpretation requires knowledge of normal anatomy

1. Intraoral Radiographs

a. Periapical Radiographs

Used to evaluate:

- Root morphology
- Periapical pathology
- Periodontal ligament space
- Lamina dura

Example:

A periapical radiolucency associated with a non-vital tooth suggests apical periodontitis.

b. Bitewing Radiographs

Primarily used for:

- Interproximal caries detection

- Alveolar crest bone level evaluation

Early proximal lesions may not be clinically visible but appear as radiolucent triangles on bitewings.

c. Occlusal Radiographs

Used for:

- Localization of impacted teeth
- Salivary stones
- Jaw expansion

Interpretation Considerations

Radiographic interpretation must consider:

- Projection geometry
- Superimposition
- Artifacts
- Contrast and density

A radiolucent area does not automatically indicate pathology. For example, the mental foramen may mimic periapical pathology if not properly identified.

III. Digital Radiography

Digital systems provide:

- Reduced radiation exposure
- Image enhancement
- Immediate viewing
- Storage and transmission capabilities

Contrast adjustment and magnification can enhance diagnostic accuracy but may also introduce interpretation bias.

IV. Panoramic Radiography

Panoramic imaging offers a broad overview of:

- Maxilla and mandible
- Impacted teeth
- Developmental anomalies

- Jaw lesions

Limitations include distortion and reduced resolution compared to intraoral radiographs.

Example:

Impacted third molars with proximity to the inferior alveolar canal are first identified on panoramic imaging before further assessment.

V. Cone-Beam Computed Tomography (CBCT)

CBCT provides three-dimensional imaging and has transformed dental diagnostics.

Indications

- Implant planning
- Impacted teeth localization
- Endodontic complex anatomy
- Root fractures
- Pathology assessment
- TMJ evaluation

Advantages

- 3D visualization
- Accurate measurements
- Elimination of superimposition

Limitations

- Higher radiation dose than intraoral radiographs
- Artifact presence
- Interpretation complexity

Clinical Example

A mandibular molar with persistent symptoms despite root canal therapy may show a missed MB2 canal on CBCT not visible on periapical radiograph.

VI. Adjunctive Diagnostic Aids

1. Caries Detection Technologies

- Laser fluorescence devices
- Transillumination
- Quantitative light-induced fluorescence

These tools detect early demineralization but require correlation with clinical findings.

2. Periodontal Diagnostic Aids

- Microbial testing
- Genetic susceptibility markers
- Salivary biomarkers

Such tests supplement but do not replace clinical examination.

3. Pulpal Blood Flow Assessment

Laser Doppler flowmetry assesses vascular supply rather than neural response, potentially more accurate than traditional vitality tests.

4. Oral Cancer Screening Adjuncts

Light-based detection devices may enhance visualization of suspicious lesions but do not replace biopsy.

VII. Interpretation: The Art and Science

Interpretation requires:

- Pattern recognition
- Differential diagnosis formulation
- Correlation with history
- Risk assessment integration

For example, a radiolucent lesion at the apex of a vital tooth requires reconsideration of diagnosis—perhaps a non-odontogenic cyst rather than periapical pathology.

VIII. Diagnostic Errors

Errors may arise from:

- Observer bias
- Incomplete examination
- Overreliance on imaging

- Failure to correlate findings

False positives can lead to overtreatment; false negatives may delay necessary care.

IX. Case-Based Illustrations

Case 1: Deep Caries

Clinical: Large occlusal cavity

Radiograph: Approaching pulp

Test: Lingering cold response

Diagnosis: Irreversible pulpitis

Case 2: Implant Planning

Clinical: Missing mandibular first molar

Panoramic: Adequate bone height

CBCT: Lingual undercut detected

Treatment modified to prevent perforation.

X. Radiation Safety

The ALARA principle (As Low As Reasonably Achievable) governs radiographic exposure. Indications must justify imaging.

Lead aprons, thyroid collars, and digital sensors reduce risk.

XI. Medico-Legal Implications

Failure to obtain appropriate imaging before treatment may constitute negligence. Conversely, excessive or unjustified imaging may also raise ethical concerns.

Proper documentation must include:

- Indication for imaging
- Interpretation notes
- Correlation with clinical findings

For example, failure to detect a periapical lesion visible on radiograph that later results in infection may be scrutinized legally.

Comparative Matrix: Diagnostic Tools and Imaging in Dentistry:

Modality	**Dimensional Output**	**Primary Indications**	**Advantages**	**Limitations**	**Radiation Level**	**Clinical Example**
Clinical Examination	Direct visual/ tactile	Caries, fractures, periodontal disease, mucosal lesions	Non-invasive, immediate, no radiation	Limited to visible surfaces; subjective	None	Detecting incipient white spot lesion
Pulp Vitality Testing	Functional response	Pulpal status assessment	Simple, inexpensive	Neural response ≠ vascular health	None	Lingering cold response → irreversible pulpitis
Periapical Radiograph	2D	Periapical pathology, root morphology	High resolution for apices	Superimposition, distortion	Low	Apical radiolucency in necrotic tooth
Bitewing Radiograph	2D	Interproximal caries, crestal bone	Best for proximal decay detection	No apical visualization	Low	Early proximal caries detection

Occlusal Radiograph	2D	Impacted teeth, sialoliths	Broader field than PA	Limited fine detail	Low – Moderate	Localization of supernumerary tooth
Panoramic Radiograph	2D (broad view)	Impacted teeth, jaw pathology, development	Large coverage area	Lower resolution, distortion	Moderate	Third molar proximity to canal
CBCT (Cone-Beam CT)	3D	Implant planning, fractures, complex anatomy	Accurate spatial analysis, no superimposition	Higher dose, artifact risk	Moderate – High (varies by FOV)	Evaluating bone width before implant
Digital Radiography	2D	Routine intraoral imaging	Reduced radiation, image enhancement	Potential over-enhancement bias	Low	Monitoring bone levels digitally
Laser Fluorescence (Caries	Quantitative reading	Early enamel demineralizatio	Detects non-cavitated	False positives (stains,	None	Occlusal early caries detecti

Detection)		n	lesions	calculus)		on
Transillumination (FOTI/NIRI)	Optical visualization	Interproximal caries, cracks	No radiation	Limited depth penetration	None	Crack detection in anterior teeth
Periodontal Probing	Measurement (mm)	Attachment loss assessment	Objective measurement	Technique sensitive	None	6 mm pocket depth evaluation
Microbial/Salivary Tests	Biochemical analysis	Periodontal risk, caries risk	Risk stratification	Adjunctive only	None	High Streptococcus mutans count
Oral Cancer Adjunct Devices	Light-based tissue visualization	Suspicious mucosal lesions	Enhances visualization	Does not replace biopsy	None	Persistent leukoplakic lesion

Treatment Planning Strategies

Dr. C. Chandra Lekha
M.D.S (Orthodontics & Dentofacial Orthopedics)
Dr. Chandra's Dental & Orthodontic Care
Madurai, Tamil Nadu, India

Sequencing, prioritization, phased treatment planning, and prognosis assessment.

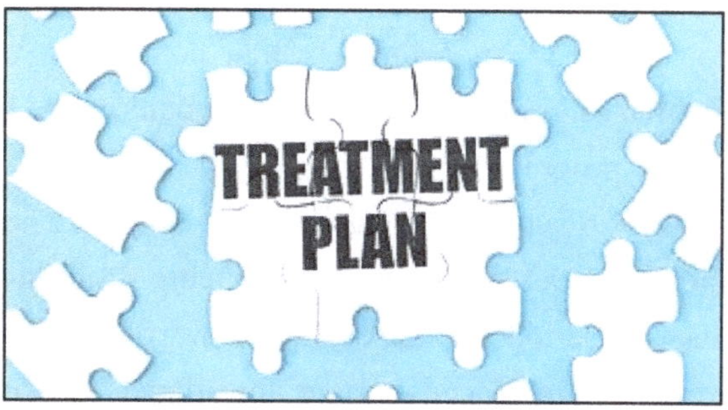

Treatment planning in dentistry is an intellectual and ethical process that transforms diagnostic findings into a structured roadmap of care. It is neither a mechanical listing of procedures nor a purely technical exercise; rather, it represents a dynamic synthesis of diagnosis, risk assessment, patient-centered goals, biological feasibility, and long-term maintenance considerations. Effective treatment planning requires strategic sequencing, thoughtful prioritization, phased execution, and continuous prognosis evaluation. These elements operate within a probability-based framework, acknowledging that dental outcomes are influenced by biological variability, patient compliance, systemic conditions, and technical factors.

Sequencing refers to the logical order in which interventions are delivered to maximize therapeutic success and minimize complications. Biological principles dictate that disease control precedes definitive rehabilitation. Acute conditions are addressed first, followed by stabilization of the oral environment, and finally by definitive restorative or prosthetic reconstruction. For example, in a patient presenting with multiple carious lesions, generalized moderate periodontitis, and missing posterior teeth, immediate placement of fixed prostheses without addressing periodontal inflammation would jeopardize long-term success. Proper sequencing requires initial management of pain or infection, followed by periodontal therapy and caries control, before definitive restorative rehabilitation is undertaken. This biologically oriented progression ensures that definitive procedures are placed into a stable, healthy environment.

Prioritization involves determining which conditions require urgent attention and which can be deferred. Urgency is determined by severity of symptoms, risk of progression, systemic implications, and potential for irreversible damage. A symptomatic irreversible pulpitis takes precedence over replacement of a defective but asymptomatic restoration. Similarly, rapidly progressing periodontal disease may warrant early intervention before elective cosmetic procedures are considered. Prioritization must also account for patient-centered factors, including financial constraints, time availability, esthetic expectations, and psychological readiness. In certain cases, a patient may prioritize anterior esthetics over posterior occlusal rehabilitation. While the clinician must educate the patient regarding biological risks, collaborative prioritization enhances adherence and shared decision-making.

Phased treatment planning structures care into organized stages that reflect disease control, stabilization, rehabilitation, and maintenance. The emergency phase addresses acute pain, infection, trauma, or other urgent concerns. The disease control phase focuses on elimination of active pathology through caries removal, endodontic therapy, periodontal treatment, and risk factor modification. The definitive phase includes prosthodontic reconstruction, implant placement, orthodontics, or advanced restorative procedures. Finally, the maintenance phase emphasizes long-term monitoring, preventive care, and reinforcement of oral hygiene practices. Phased planning recognizes that complex cases evolve over time and that biological responses to earlier interventions may influence subsequent decisions.

Consider a patient with advanced attrition, reduced vertical dimension, generalized periodontal attachment loss, and multiple missing posterior teeth. Immediate full-mouth reconstruction without preliminary periodontal stabilization would be biologically unsound. Instead, initial periodontal therapy and occlusal analysis are performed, provisional restorations may be used to test vertical dimension changes, and definitive prostheses are fabricated only after functional stability is achieved. This phased approach reduces risk and allows reassessment at each stage, reinforcing the principle that treatment planning is iterative rather than static.

Prognosis assessment is central to strategic planning. Each tooth, quadrant, and overall dentition must be assigned a short-term and long-term prognosis based on structural integrity, periodontal support, endodontic status, occlusal forces, and patient-related risk factors such as smoking or diabetes. Prognosis is not an absolute prediction but a probability estimate grounded in evidence and clinical experience. For example, a molar with severe furcation involvement and Grade III mobility may carry a questionable or poor prognosis despite successful endodontic therapy. Conversely, a structurally compromised tooth with adequate ferrule and controlled periodontal conditions may have a favorable outlook following restoration.

Prognosis assessment guides whether teeth are retained, extracted, or used as abutments. In prosthodontic planning, abutment selection depends on load distribution, periodontal health, crown-root ratio, and anticipated occlusal forces. Retaining a tooth with poor prognosis as a fixed bridge abutment may compromise the entire prosthesis. Thus, prognosis evaluation must extend beyond individual teeth to encompass functional units and biomechanical considerations.

Strategic treatment planning also requires anticipation of complications and long-term maintenance demands. Implant therapy, for instance, may demonstrate high survival rates in healthy individuals but reduced success in smokers or poorly controlled diabetics. In such patients, risk modification and informed consent become integral components of planning. Similarly, extensive adhesive restorations in high caries risk patients may require aggressive preventive protocols before definitive placement.

Occlusion and functional harmony represent additional dimensions of planning strategy. In cases involving full-mouth rehabilitation, diagnostic wax-ups, mounted casts, and provisional restorations allow simulation of occlusal changes before definitive treatment. This diagnostic phase provides insight into esthetics, phonetics, temporomandibular joint response, and patient adaptation. Through this process, treatment becomes a carefully staged progression rather than an irreversible leap.

Interdisciplinary coordination often defines complex treatment strategies. Orthodontic, periodontal, endodontic, and prosthodontic therapies may need integration. For example, orthodontic extrusion may be required to enhance ferrule before crown placement. Periodontal crown lengthening may precede restorative procedures. Implant site development through bone grafting may be necessary prior to prosthetic planning. Effective sequencing ensures that each discipline contributes optimally without compromising others.

Economic considerations inevitably influence planning strategies. Ideal treatment recommendations must be balanced with patient affordability and willingness. Ethical practice demands presentation of evidence-based alternatives with transparent discussion of risks and benefits. A staged approach may allow patients to distribute financial commitments over time while still achieving biologically sound outcomes.

Reevaluation forms a critical component of phased planning. After disease control measures are completed, clinical parameters must be reassessed before proceeding to definitive care. Periodontal pocket reduction, improved oral hygiene indices, and stabilized occlusion signal readiness for restorative phases. If disease persists, modification of strategy is necessary. Thus, treatment planning is responsive to clinical outcomes rather than rigidly predetermined.

The dynamic nature of prognosis further emphasizes the need for continuous reassessment. A tooth initially classified as questionable may demonstrate improvement following periodontal therapy and become suitable for restoration. Conversely, deterioration in systemic health may alter the prognosis of previously stable implants or teeth. Strategic planning incorporates flexibility, allowing adaptation to evolving biological realities.

From a medico-legal perspective, comprehensive documentation of sequencing rationale, prognosis estimation, and alternative options discussed is essential. Failure to phase treatment appropriately or to inform patients of questionable prognoses may expose clinicians to allegations of overtreatment or negligence. Transparent communication regarding uncertainty strengthens both patient trust and professional accountability.

In essence, treatment planning strategies represent the intellectual architecture of dental care. Sequencing ensures biological coherence, prioritization addresses urgency and patient-centered goals, phased planning structures complexity into manageable stages, and prognosis assessment anchors decisions in probability-based reasoning. Together, these principles transform diagnostic information into structured, ethical, and sustainable therapeutic action.

Integrated Treatment Planning Matrix:

Strategic Component	Definition & Purpose	Clinical Example	Prognostic Consideration	Clinical Tips for Practice
Emergency Phase	Immediate management of pain, infection, trauma, or	Patient presents with acute apical abscess	Short-term stabilization improves systemic	Always relieve pain first; document baseline

	acute pathology to stabilize the patient	and facial swelling → incision and drainage + initiation of endodontic therapy	and local prognosis before definitive care	symptoms; reassess vitality after emergency pulp therapy
Disease Control Phase	Elimination of active disease processes (caries, periodontal inflammation, endodontic infection)	Generalized bleeding on probing and multiple carious lesions → scaling and root planing + caries excavation	Periodontal stabilization improves survival of future restorations and prostheses	Avoid placing definitive crowns before inflammation control; reassess plaque indices before moving forward
Stabilization Phase	Establish structural and functional stability prior to complex rehabilitation	Placement of provisional restorations to test vertical dimension in severe attrition case	Functional adaptation determines long-term occlusal prognosis	Use long-term provisionals to evaluate esthetics, phonetics, and TMJ response
Definitive Restorativ	Final prosthetic	Implant placement	Implant survival	Confirm bone quality

e Phase	or restorative reconstruction after disease control	after bone graft healing	influenced by systemic factors (smoking, diabetes)	radiographically; ensure patient compliance before implant surgery
Maintenance Phase	Long-term monitoring and prevention to sustain treatment outcomes	Periodontal recall every 3–4 months after therapy	Maintenance compliance directly affects tooth survival probability	Customize recall interval based on risk level, not a universal 6-month rule
Prioritization Strategy	Determining urgency and biological risk before elective procedures	Symptomatic irreversible pulpitis treated before cosmetic veneers	Untreated pulpal pathology compromises overall prognosis	Address biologic threats before esthetic enhancements
Sequencing Logic	Ordering interventions to prevent procedural interference	Orthodontic alignment before definitive prosthodontic crowns	Improper sequence may require crown removal later	Always consider whether future therapy will alter current restorations
Tooth-Level Prognosis Assessme	Evaluating structural integrity, periodontal	Molar with Grade III furcation	Poor abutment choice may	Avoid using teeth with guarded prognosis as

nt	support, endodontic status	involvement → questionable prognosis	jeopardize fixed bridge	key abutments
Systemic Risk Integration	Incorporating systemic health into planning	Poorly controlled diabetic patient requiring implant	Increased peri-implantitis risk	Coordinate with physician; optimize glycemic control before surgery
Financial Phasing Strategy	Structuring treatment according to patient affordability without compromising biology	Staged quadrant dentistry over multiple visits	Delays may affect disease progression	Clearly explain risks of postponement; document patient decisions
Interdisciplinary Coordination	Sequencing across specialties for optimal outcome	Crown lengthening before final crown placement	Insufficient ferrule compromises crown survival	Evaluate biologic width before restorative preparation
Reevaluation Checkpoint	Reassessing outcomes before progressing to next phase	Re-probing pockets after scaling before crown fabrication	Persistent inflammation lowers restorative longevity	Never skip reassessment appointment before definitive prosthetics

Managing Dental Caries

Dr. Ravi Gupta
Associate Professor,
Department of Conservative Dentistry and Endodontics,
Manipal University College Malaysia (MUCM),
Jalan Batu Hampar, Bukit Baru, 75150
Melaka, Malaysia

Decision-making for prevention, remineralization, restorations, and minimally invasive care.

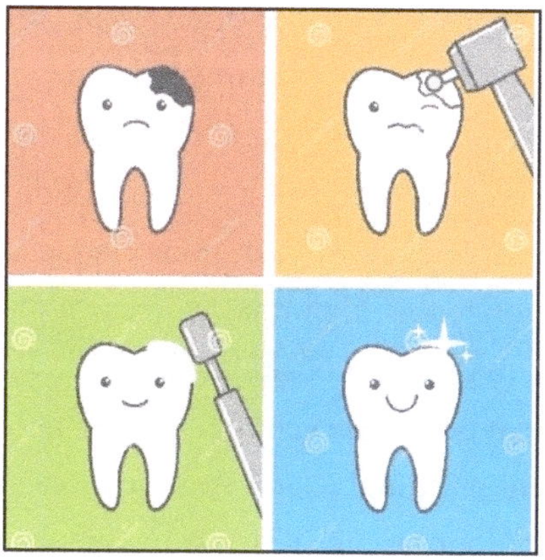

Dental caries remains one of the most prevalent chronic diseases worldwide, yet contemporary understanding has shifted dramatically from a purely surgical model toward a biologically informed, risk-based, minimally invasive philosophy. Caries is no longer conceptualized as an inevitable consequence of sugar exposure requiring mechanical removal of affected tissue; rather, it is understood as a dynamic, biofilm-mediated, diet-modulated disease characterized by cycles of demineralization and remineralization. Effective management, therefore, requires strategic decision-making grounded in disease activity assessment, patient risk profiling, lesion staging, and long-term behavioral modification. The modern clinician's role extends beyond restoring cavities to controlling disease processes and preserving tooth structure whenever biologically feasible. The pathogenesis of dental caries involves complex interactions among fermentable carbohydrates, acidogenic and aciduric bacteria, host susceptibility, saliva composition, and time. Acid production from bacterial metabolism leads to subsurface enamel demineralization. However, this process is reversible during early stages if protective factors such as fluoride exposure, adequate salivary flow, and dietary modification are introduced. Thus, management decisions hinge on identifying whether a lesion is active or arrested, cavitated or non-cavitated, and whether the patient's overall risk environment supports non-operative intervention.

Risk assessment constitutes the intellectual foundation of caries management. Caries risk is determined by evaluating past caries experience, oral hygiene status, fluoride exposure, dietary habits, salivary function, socioeconomic factors, and systemic conditions. A patient with multiple new lesions over the past year, poor plaque control, and frequent sugar intake is categorized as high risk, whereas a patient with no recent caries and stable oral hygiene is considered low risk. Risk status influences both the intensity and type of intervention. For example, in a low-risk adult with a single incipient proximal lesion confined to enamel, non-operative management may be appropriate. In contrast, the same lesion in a high-risk adolescent may warrant more aggressive preventive measures and closer monitoring.

Prevention remains the primary strategy in caries management. Fluoride therapy enhances enamel remineralization and inhibits bacterial metabolism. Topical fluoride varnishes, high-fluoride toothpaste, and professionally applied gels are indicated in moderate- to high-risk patients. Dietary counseling is equally critical. Frequent consumption of fermentable carbohydrates increases acid challenges, prolonging demineralization periods. Educating patients regarding frequency rather than merely quantity of sugar intake can substantially alter disease trajectory. Salivary stimulation through sugar-free chewing gum or management of xerostomia in medically compromised patients further supports remineralization.

A clinical example illustrates the preventive paradigm. A 12-year-old patient presents with multiple chalky white spot lesions on the buccal surfaces of maxillary incisors. These lesions are non-cavitated and demonstrate surface roughness consistent with activity. Rather than preparing and restoring each lesion, the clinician institutes fluoride varnish applications every three months, provides dietary counseling, and reinforces oral hygiene. After six months, the lesions exhibit a smoother, shinier surface, indicating arrest. No surgical intervention was required, and tooth structure was preserved. This example underscores the importance of recognizing caries as a reversible process during early stages. Remineralization strategies extend beyond fluoride alone. Casein phosphopeptide-amorphous calcium phosphate (CPP-ACP), bioactive glass materials, and other calcium-phosphate–based technologies aim to enhance mineral deposition. While evidence varies in strength, these adjunctive agents may be useful in selected patients with high demineralization activity. The decision to employ such therapies should be evidence-informed and tailored to individual risk.

Sealant application represents another preventive modality, particularly in pediatric and adolescent populations. Occlusal pits and fissures are anatomically predisposed to plaque retention. Application of resin-based or glass ionomer sealants creates a physical barrier that prevents bacterial colonization. In moderate-risk children, sealing deep fissures without evidence of cavitation may prevent future operative treatment. Even in cases of early non-cavitated occlusal lesions, sealants may arrest progression by cutting off nutrient supply to bacteria.

When lesions progress beyond the threshold of remineralization and cavitation occurs, restorative intervention becomes necessary. However, the modern operative philosophy emphasizes minimally invasive dentistry. This approach prioritizes maximal preservation of healthy tooth structure, selective caries removal, and adhesive restorative materials. Historically, complete removal of all softened dentin was advocated to eliminate infection. Contemporary evidence indicates that in deep lesions approaching the pulp, selective removal of infected dentin while preserving affected dentin reduces risk of pulpal exposure and maintains vitality.

Consider a 35-year-old patient with a deep occlusal carious lesion in a mandibular molar. Radiographically, the lesion approximates the pulp, yet vitality testing indicates reversible pulpitis. Instead of aggressive excavation that risks pulp exposure, the clinician performs selective caries removal, leaving firm but leathery dentin over the pulpal floor, and restores the tooth with a bonded composite restoration. The sealed environment deprives residual bacteria of nutrients, reducing their activity. Long-term follow-up demonstrates pulpal health and absence of symptoms. This case exemplifies biologically respectful intervention.

Material selection in restorative management must reflect caries risk, moisture control, lesion location, and esthetic demands. Resin composites provide excellent esthetics and adhesive bonding but require meticulous isolation. Glass ionomer cements offer fluoride release and chemical adhesion, making them advantageous in high-risk patients or situations with limited moisture control. The decision is not purely material-based but contextual, integrating patient factors and lesion characteristics.

Minimally invasive techniques such as atraumatic restorative treatment (ART) and silver diamine fluoride (SDF) application further expand non-traditional options. ART employs hand instruments and high-viscosity glass ionomer to manage caries in settings where conventional rotary instrumentation may be impractical. SDF arrests caries by exerting antimicrobial and remineralizing effects, though it results in black staining of arrested lesions. In elderly or medically compromised patients unable to tolerate extensive procedures, SDF offers a pragmatic solution to control disease progression without surgical excavation.

The decision to restore rather than remineralize is determined by lesion depth, cavitation status, cleansability, and patient compliance. A non-cavitated interproximal enamel lesion may be monitored with fluoride therapy and radiographic follow-up. However, once dentinal involvement compromises structural integrity or plaque control becomes impossible due to cavitation, restoration is indicated. The threshold for operative intervention must balance risk of progression against risk of overtreatment. Long-term management requires reassessment and maintenance. Caries is a chronic disease with episodic activity. Restorations do not cure caries; they repair structural damage. Without modification of risk factors, recurrent caries may develop at restoration margins. Therefore, recall intervals should be individualized based on risk. High-risk patients may require three- to four-month recall visits, while low-risk individuals may be monitored annually.

Behavioral modification is often the most challenging yet critical component of caries management. Motivational interviewing techniques can enhance patient engagement and adherence. Rather than dictating instructions, clinicians can collaborate with patients to identify achievable dietary or hygiene changes. For example, reducing sugary beverage intake from five times daily to once daily may significantly alter caries risk.

Caries management in special populations introduces additional complexity. In pediatric patients, primary teeth require consideration of exfoliation timelines, behavior management, and parental involvement. In geriatric patients, root caries becomes prevalent due to gingival recession and reduced salivary flow. Management strategies must adapt to these biological realities. For instance, application of high-fluoride toothpaste and SDF may be particularly effective in elderly patients with limited dexterity.

The integration of diagnostic technologies enhances decision-making. Bitewing radiographs assist in detecting proximal lesions not visible clinically. Laser fluorescence devices may aid in identifying occlusal demineralization. However, interpretation must be cautious to avoid false positives leading to unnecessary restorations. Diagnostic findings should always be correlated with clinical assessment and risk status.

Ethical considerations permeate caries management decisions.

Overtreatment through restoration of non-cavitated lesions contradicts minimally invasive principles, while undertreatment of active dentinal lesions risks pulpal involvement. Transparent communication regarding options, benefits, risks, and uncertainties is essential. Patients should understand that non-operative management requires adherence and monitoring, whereas operative treatment addresses structural damage but does not eliminate disease susceptibility.

A comprehensive example illustrates integrated decision-making. A 28-year-old patient presents with moderate caries risk, two non-cavitated proximal enamel lesions, one cavitated occlusal dentinal lesion, and frequent snacking habits. The management plan includes dietary counseling, fluoride varnish application, monitoring of enamel lesions, and minimally invasive restoration of the cavitated lesion with adhesive composite. Six months later, no progression is observed in the enamel lesions, and the patient reports reduced snacking frequency. This blended approach demonstrates prevention, remineralization, and restoration functioning cohesively. The philosophy of caries management thus embodies a shift from surgical repair to medical disease control. Decision-making is guided by lesion activity, risk assessment, structural integrity, and patient cooperation. Prevention and remineralization are prioritized whenever biologically feasible, and operative intervention is reserved for situations where structural compromise or cleansability limitations necessitate restoration. Minimally invasive techniques aim to preserve pulp vitality and tooth longevity.

Ultimately, managing dental caries requires continuous reassessment and adaptability. As patient behaviors evolve and risk profiles change, treatment strategies must be recalibrated. The goal is not merely to eliminate cavities but to maintain oral health stability through biologically sound, patient-centered, evidence-based care.

Clinical Tip Didactic Table

Managing Dental Caries: Prevention, Remineralization, Restorative Thresholds, and Minimally Invasive Care

Clinical Scenario	Diagnostic Clue	Decision Pathway	Evidence-Based Rationale	Practical Clinical Tip
Chalky white spot lesion on smooth surface	Non-cavitated, rough when dried	Remineralization protocol	Early enamel lesions are reversible	Dry the tooth before assessment; rough matte surface indicates activity
Shiny white/brown lesion	Hard, glossy surface	Monitor, no operative care	Arrested lesions do not require restoration	Do not restore color changes alone; assess texture and activity
Proximal enamel lesion on bitewing	Radiolucency limited to enamel	Fluoride + dietary modification + 6-month review	Many enamel lesions can remineralize	Use risk status to decide recall interval
Deep occlusal fissure in child	No radiographic dentin involvement	Sealant placement	Sealants prevent bacterial colonization	Etch thoroughly; check isolation before curing
Cavitate	Explorer	Minimally	Cavitation	Remove

d dentinal lesion	catch + radiographic dentin involvement	invasive restoration	prevents effective plaque control	infected dentin selectively; avoid over-preparation
Deep caries near pulp	Radiolucency approaching pulp + reversible pulpitis	Selective caries removal	Preserves pulp vitality	Leave firm dentin over pulp; avoid pulp exposure if possible
High caries risk patient	Multiple new lesions in past year	Intensive preventive program	Disease control before repeated restorations	Prescribe high-fluoride toothpaste (5,000 ppm) when indicated
Xerostomic patient	Dry mucosa, root caries	Saliva substitutes + fluoride + diet control	Saliva deficiency increases demineralization	Recommend sugar-free gum with xylitol for salivary stimulation
Elderly	Soft	Glass	Fluoride	Consider

root caries	cervical lesion	ionomer or SDF	release beneficial	SDF if isolation difficult or patient medically compromised
Recurrent caries at restoration margin	Marginal staining + softness	Repair if localized, replace if extensive	Preservation of sound structure preferred	Explore margins gently; not all staining is recurrent decay
High esthetic demand anterior lesion	Small proximal lesion	Resin infiltration or micro-invasive approach	Avoid aggressive preparation	Consider resin infiltration for early proximal lesions
Pediatric patient with poor cooperation	Multiple cavitated primary teeth	Atraumatic restorative treatment	Minimally invasive + fluoride release	Hand instruments may reduce anxiety and need for anesthesia
Frequent sugary beverage	Dietary history reveals	Behavioral counseling	Frequency more important	Use motivational

intake	high frequency		than quantity	interviewing instead of lecturing
Moderate-risk adult	Isolated lesion, good hygiene	Combined preventive + conservative restoration	Tailored care reduces overtreatment	Avoid "drill-first" approach in moderate risk
Arrested occlusal lesion	Dark, hard fissure	Monitor	Hardness indicates inactivity	Do not restore based on discoloration alone

Lesion Activity Assessment Guide

Parameter	Active Lesion	Arrested Lesion	Clinical Teaching Note
Surface texture	Rough	Smooth	Always air dry before tactile evaluation
Appearance	Matte, opaque	Shiny	Visual inspection under good lighting essential
Plaque stagnation area	Often present	May be absent	Location influences risk
Progression risk	High	Low	Monitor rather than restore if arrested

Restorative Threshold Decision Table

Lesion Depth	Cavitation	Risk Status	Recommended Action
Enamel only	No	Low	Monitor + fluoride
Enamel only	No	High	Intensive remineralization
Outer dentin	No cavitation	Moderate	Preventive + close review
Dentin with cavitation	Yes	Any	Minimally invasive restoration
Deep dentin near pulp	Yes	Controlled risk	Selective caries removal

Minimally Invasive Material Selection Table

Clinical Condition	Preferred Material	Why	Tip
High caries risk	Glass ionomer	Fluoride release	Ideal for cervical lesions
Esthetic zone	Resin composite	Superior esthetics	Ensure strict isolation
Moisture control difficult	Glass ionomer	Chemical adhesion	Avoid desiccation
Deep lesion near pulp	Bioactive liner + composite	Pulp protection	Avoid calcium hydroxide unless indicated
Non-	Silver diamine	Arrests	Inform patient

restorable but arrestable lesion	fluoride	progression	about black staining

Recall and Monitoring Strategy Table

Risk Category	Recall Interval	Radiographic Interval	Preventive Focus
Low	12 months	18–24 months	Maintenance hygiene
Moderate	6 months	12–18 months	Fluoride reinforcement
High	3–4 months	6–12 months	Intensive disease control

Didactic Core Teaching Principles

Principle	Clinical Meaning
Caries is a disease, not a hole	Treat cause before consequence
Activity determines action	Not all lesions need drilling
Risk modifies threshold	High-risk patients require earlier intervention
Preserve tooth structure	Adhesive dentistry supports minimal removal
Restoration is not cure	Behavior modification prevents recurrence

Periodontal Decision Pathways

Dr. Vinita Dahiya
Reader
Periodontist & Oral Implantologist
Consultant, Physiodent Dental & Wellness Clinic, West Delhi

When to observe, nonsurgical therapy, surgical intervention, and maintenance planning.

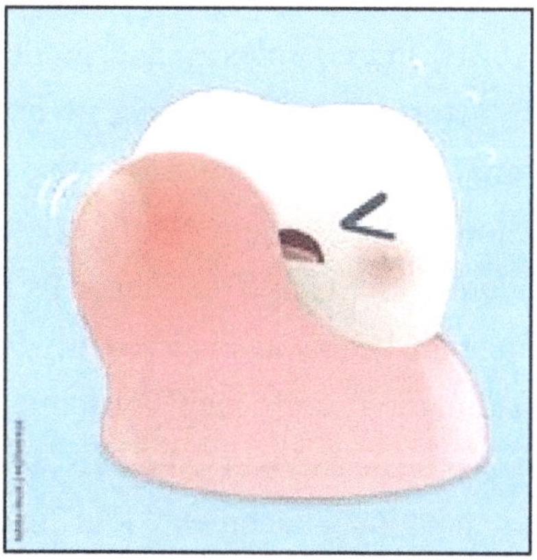

Periodontal disease represents a chronic inflammatory condition initiated by microbial biofilm and modified by host response, systemic health, and environmental factors. Its management is not defined by a single intervention but by a structured decision pathway that moves from diagnosis to risk assessment, disease control, potential surgical correction, and long-term maintenance. Effective periodontal care requires disciplined sequencing, calibrated prognosis assessment, and ongoing reassessment.

The clinician must determine when observation is sufficient, when nonsurgical therapy is indicated, when surgical intervention becomes necessary, and how maintenance strategies sustain stability over time. These decisions are rooted in contemporary classification frameworks, particularly those outlined in the 2017 World Workshop on the

Classification of Periodontal and Peri-Implant Diseases and Conditions, jointly organized by the American Academy of Periodontology and the European Federation of Periodontology. This staging and grading system provides structure for severity assessment and risk estimation, thereby informing therapeutic pathways.

Periodontal decision-making begins with comprehensive evaluation. Diagnosis requires measurement of probing depths, clinical attachment loss, bleeding on probing, plaque levels, mobility, furcation involvement, mucogingival status, and radiographic bone levels. These data allow staging based on severity and complexity and grading based on rate of progression and risk factors such as smoking or uncontrolled diabetes. However, staging alone does not dictate treatment; disease activity and patient-specific risk modify decisions.

For example, a patient with Stage II periodontitis but excellent plaque control and no bleeding may be managed differently from a similar patient with persistent inflammation and high systemic risk. Observation represents a valid management pathway when disease is absent, inactive, or stable. Gingivitis without attachment loss may resolve through improved oral hygiene alone. In such cases, professional prophylaxis combined with patient education may suffice. Similarly, a patient with historical attachment loss but no current bleeding or pocket progression may be considered stable and maintained without escalation to surgical therapy. The decision to observe is not passive neglect but active monitoring. Documentation of baseline measurements and scheduled reevaluation are critical components. Observation is particularly appropriate in low-risk patients with shallow probing depths and minimal inflammation. It reflects an understanding that overtreatment carries risks, including unnecessary tissue removal, cost, and patient morbidity.

Nonsurgical periodontal therapy forms the cornerstone of active disease management. Scaling and root planing aim to disrupt subgingival biofilm, remove calculus, and reduce bacterial load. Adjunctive measures may include local antimicrobial agents, systemic antibiotics in selected cases, and reinforcement of oral hygiene instruction. The decision to initiate nonsurgical therapy is generally indicated when probing depths exceed physiologic limits, bleeding on probing persists, or radiographic bone loss is present in conjunction with clinical inflammation. Nonsurgical therapy addresses the etiologic factor—microbial plaque—while also modifying the host inflammatory response through mechanical debridement.

Clinical evidence consistently demonstrates that thorough nonsurgical therapy can significantly reduce probing depths and improve clinical attachment levels, particularly in pockets of moderate depth. For example, a patient presenting with generalized 5 to 6 mm pockets and bleeding on probing may exhibit reduction to 3 to 4 mm pockets following comprehensive scaling and root planing combined with improved plaque control. Reevaluation at four to eight weeks determines whether residual pockets persist. The concept of reevaluation is central to periodontal decision pathways; treatment is not considered complete until the biological response is assessed.

If inflammation resolves and pocket depths are reduced to maintainable levels, surgical intervention may be unnecessary. However, nonsurgical therapy has limitations. Deep pockets with complex anatomy, furcation involvement, vertical bone defects, or residual calculus inaccessible to instrumentation may not respond fully. When residual probing depths remain greater than 5 or 6 mm with persistent bleeding after initial therapy, surgical intervention may be considered. The decision to proceed surgically is based on the goal of achieving improved access for debridement, reducing pocket depth, and creating a maintainable architecture. Surgical options range from open flap debridement to resective procedures and regenerative techniques. The choice depends on defect morphology, systemic health, esthetic considerations, and patient preference.

For example, in a mandibular molar with Grade II furcation involvement and persistent 7 mm pockets after nonsurgical therapy, surgical access may permit visualization and debridement not achievable through closed instrumentation. In cases of vertical intrabony defects, regenerative procedures employing bone grafts and barrier membranes may aim to restore lost attachment. Yet surgical therapy is not universally indicated for all deep pockets. The clinician must evaluate whether anticipated benefits outweigh risks, including postoperative morbidity and cost. Additionally, patient compliance plays a decisive role. Surgical intervention without adequate plaque control may yield limited benefit.

Maintenance planning represents the final and ongoing stage of periodontal decision pathways. Periodontitis is a chronic condition characterized by episodic exacerbations. Even after successful active therapy, susceptibility persists. Periodontal maintenance, sometimes termed supportive periodontal therapy, involves regular reassessment of probing depths, reinforcement of oral hygiene, removal of biofilm and calculus, and monitoring of systemic and behavioral risk factors. Maintenance intervals are individualized based on risk assessment. High-risk patients, including smokers or those with poorly controlled diabetes, may require three-month recalls, whereas low-risk stable patients may be maintained at longer intervals.

The importance of maintenance cannot be overstated. Longitudinal studies demonstrate that patients who adhere to regular supportive therapy exhibit significantly lower rates of tooth loss compared to those who do not. Maintenance is not merely prophylaxis; it is a structured continuation of periodontal care. Failure to maintain supportive therapy may lead to recurrence of inflammation and progression of attachment loss, potentially negating benefits achieved during active treatment.

Decision pathways in periodontology also integrate systemic health considerations. Diabetes, smoking, immunosuppression, and genetic predisposition modify host response and influence both disease progression and treatment outcomes. A patient with poorly controlled diabetes may exhibit exaggerated inflammatory response and delayed healing. In such cases, coordination with medical providers to improve glycemic control becomes part of periodontal management. The decision to proceed with surgery may be deferred until systemic parameters stabilize. Conversely, a non-smoking patient with well-controlled systemic health may respond favorably to nonsurgical therapy alone.

Patient-centered factors further influence decision pathways. Financial constraints, anxiety, esthetic concerns, and expectations shape acceptance of recommended therapies. Transparent communication regarding benefits, limitations, and alternatives is essential. For instance, a patient with localized advanced bone loss may elect extraction and implant placement instead of regenerative surgery. The clinician must present evidence-based options without coercion, ensuring informed consent and realistic expectations. Prognosis assessment intersects with each stage of the pathway. Individual tooth prognosis considers attachment level, mobility, furcation involvement, crown-to-root ratio, and restorative value. Overall periodontal prognosis reflects systemic risk, compliance, and disease severity.

Teeth with hopeless prognosis may be extracted during initial therapy to facilitate hygiene and reduce bacterial burden. Retaining severely compromised teeth without strategic benefit may hinder overall periodontal stability. However, extraction decisions must be made cautiously, balancing preservation against long-term predictability.

Reevaluation remains a recurring theme. After nonsurgical therapy, after surgery, and during maintenance, measurements are repeated and compared with baseline data. Improvement validates the chosen pathway; lack of response prompts reconsideration. For example, persistent bleeding despite adequate debridement may signal systemic contribution or patient noncompliance. Adjustments in maintenance frequency or adjunctive therapy may be required.

Ethical and medico-legal considerations permeate periodontal decision-making. Documentation of baseline findings, risk discussions, treatment rationale, and maintenance recommendations protects both patient and practitioner. Failure to diagnose or treat progressive periodontal disease may constitute negligence. Conversely, performing unnecessary surgery without clear indication may also raise ethical concerns. The clinician must justify each decision within accepted professional standards and evidence-based guidelines.

Interdisciplinary coordination frequently influences periodontal pathways. Orthodontic movement may be contraindicated in active periodontitis. Prosthodontic planning depends on periodontal stability. Implant placement requires assessment of periodontal susceptibility, as history of periodontitis increases risk of peri-implantitis. Thus, periodontal management often precedes or integrates with restorative and surgical disciplines.

Consider a comprehensive clinical example. A 50-year-old patient presents with generalized Stage III periodontitis, smoking history, and inconsistent dental visits. Initial probing reveals multiple sites of 6 to 8 mm pockets with bleeding. Radiographs demonstrate vertical bone defects in posterior sextants. The decision pathway begins with patient education, smoking cessation counseling, and comprehensive scaling and root planing. After six weeks, reevaluation shows reduction of many pockets to 4 mm but persistent 7 mm defects in two molar regions. Surgical regenerative therapy is proposed for those localized areas. Following successful healing, the patient enters a strict three-month maintenance program. Over five years, attachment levels remain stable, and no additional teeth are lost. This case illustrates sequential application of nonsurgical therapy, selective surgical intervention, and disciplined maintenance. Contrast this with a similar patient who declines maintenance visits after initial therapy. Within two years, recurrent inflammation and additional attachment loss occur. The divergence in outcomes underscores the critical role of maintenance planning within the decision pathway. Ultimately, periodontal decision pathways are iterative, evidence-informed, and patient-centered. Observation is appropriate when disease is inactive or reversible. Nonsurgical therapy addresses the microbial etiology and often suffices for moderate disease. Surgical intervention is reserved for residual defects or anatomical complexities unresponsive to conservative measures. Maintenance ensures sustainability of outcomes and mitigates recurrence. Each stage is guided by reassessment, risk evaluation, and transparent communication.

Periodontal care exemplifies the broader philosophy of modern dentistry: intervention calibrated to biological need, sequenced logically, and sustained through long-term preventive commitment. The clinician's task is not merely to reduce pocket depths but to preserve function, comfort, and oral health stability over the lifespan.

Periodontal Clinical Tip Table with Examples:

Clinical Situation	Key Diagnostic Finding	Decision Pathway	Practical Clinical Tip	Example
Localized gingivitis	Bleeding on probing, no attachment loss	Observation + oral hygiene instruction	Emphasize plaque control before scaling intensity	25-year-old with bleeding but 2–3 mm pockets improves after hygiene reinforcement
Stable reduced periodontium	Historical bone loss, no bleeding	Maintenance only	Do not overtreat stable attachment loss	60-year-old with past periodontitis but no active inflammation

				maintained at 4-month recall
Generalized 4–5 mm pockets with bleeding	Moderate inflammation	Nonsurgical therapy	Perform quadrant scaling with meticulous root planing	45-year-old smoker shows pocket reduction after SRP and improved brushing
Deep isolated 7–8 mm pocket after SRP	Persistent bleeding	Surgical access	Reevaluate 6–8 weeks post-SRP before surgery	Mandibular molar with residual deep defect treated with open flap debridement
Vertical intrabony defect	Radiographic angular bone loss	Regenerative surgery	Assess defect morphology before grafting	3-wall defect treated with bone graft and membrane

Grade II furcation involvement	Horizontal bone loss in furcation	Surgical intervention or selective odontoplasty	Furcations rarely respond completely to closed therapy	Lower molar with persistent 6 mm furcation pocket
Grade III mobility	Severe attachment loss	Evaluate prognosis for extraction	Avoid using poor-prognosis teeth as bridge abutments	Mobile molar extracted before prosthetic planning
Heavy smoker with periodontitis	Generalized inflammation + risk factor	Intensive nonsurgical + smoking cessation	Address risk factors before surgery	50-year-old reduces pocket depth after quitting smoking
Poor compliance patient	Missed recalls, plaque accumulation	Shorter maintenance interval	Maintenance success depends on adherence	3-month recall prevents recurrence
Post-surgical	Reduced pocket	Maintenance phase	Reinforce home	Regenerated molar

stable patient	depth, no bleeding		care at every visit	defect remains stable at 5-year follow-up

```
Initial Examination
   |
   ├── No attachment loss + bleeding only?
   |     └── Gingivitis → Oral hygiene instruction + prophylaxis → Reevaluate
   |
   └── Attachment loss present?
         |
         ├── Mild to Moderate pockets (4–5 mm)?
         |     └── Nonsurgical therapy (SRP) → Reevaluate 6–8 weeks
         |           |
         |           ├── Pockets reduced ≤4 mm, no bleeding?
         |           |     └── Maintenance phase
         |           |
         |           └── Persistent ≥6 mm pockets?
         |                 └── Consider surgical intervention
         |
         └── Advanced pockets (≥7 mm), vertical defects, furcation?
               └── Initial SRP → Reevaluate
                     |
                     ├── Improved?
                     |     └── Maintenance
                     └── Persistent deep defect?
                           └── Surgical therapy (access/resective/regenerative)
                                 |
                                 └── Post-surgical reevaluation → Maintenance
```

Integrated Table: Periodontal Decision Tree in Structured Clinical Format:

Stage	Clinical Findings	Decision Node	Primary Intervention	Reevaluation Criteria	Next Step	Clinical Rationale
Initial Examination	Full periodontal charting, radiographs, BOP assessment	Is attachment loss present?	Comprehensive diagnosis	Baseline probing depths, CAL, mobility	Proceed based on findings	Establish disease presence and severity
Gingival Inflammation Only	Bleeding on probing, no clinical attachment loss	No attachment loss	Oral hygiene instruction + prophylaxis	Reevaluate in 4–6 weeks	If resolved → Maintenance; if persistent → reassess compliance	Gingivitis is reversible with plaque control
Attachment Loss	Clinical attachment loss	Assess pocke	Risk stratification	PD measurements	Categorize as mild/m	Determines therape

Present	detected	t depth severity		and radiographic bone loss	oderate or advanced	utic intensity
Mild–Moderate Periodontitis	4–5 mm pockets with bleeding	Nonsurgical phase	Scaling and root planing (SRP)	Reevaluate 6–8 weeks post-SRP	If ≤4 mm and no BOP → Maintenance; if ≥6 mm persists → Surgical consideration	Majority of moderate cases respond to SRP
Post-SRP Improvement	Pocket depth ≤4 mm, no bleeding	Disease controlled	Supportive periodontal therapy	3–6 month recall	Long-term maintenance	Maintenance prevents recurrence
Post-SRP Persistent	≥6 mm pockets remain	Residual pathology	Surgical access consid	Evaluate defect morph	Surgical therapy (access	Deep sites rarely resolve

Deep Pockets			ered	ology	/resective/regenerative)	with closed therapy
Advanced Periodontitis at Baseline	≥7 mm pockets, vertical defects, furcation involvement	High disease severity	Initial SRP before surgery	Reevaluate inflammation control	If improved → Maintenance; if persistent → Surgery	Initial SRP reduces inflammation before surgical entry
Persistent Advanced Defect	Deep residual pockets with osseous defects	Surgical intervention	Access flap / resective / regenerative	Post-surgical healing review	Transition to maintenance phase	Surgery aims at access, reshaping, or regeneration
Maintenance Phase	Stable probing depths, minimal BOP	Disease stability	Supportive periodontal therapy (3–4 months)	Continuous monitoring	Modify interval based on risk	Periodontal therapy is lifelong care

Endodontic vs Extraction Decisions

Dr. Mattapudi Basavaiah Babu
Designation: Dental Officer
Dept : Conservative dentistry and endodontics
Ex- Servicemen Contributory Health Scheme Polyclinic,
Eluru, Andhra Pradesh.

Pulpal diagnosis, restorability, prognosis, retreatment, and implant considerations.

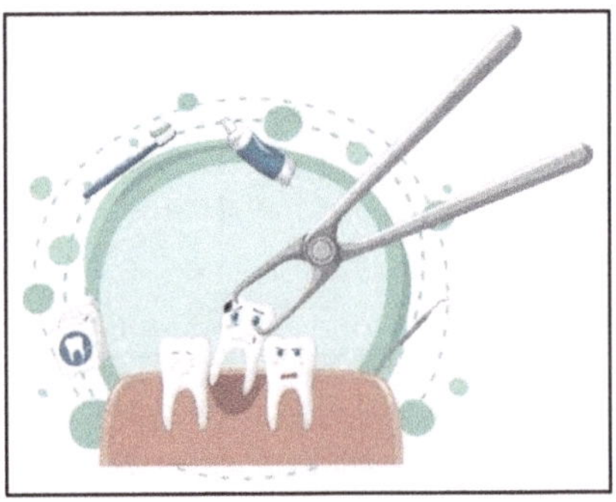

The decision between retaining a tooth through endodontic therapy and proceeding with extraction followed by prosthetic replacement represents one of the most consequential judgments in restorative dentistry. This choice is not merely technical; it integrates pulpal diagnosis, structural restorability, periodontal support, patient-specific risk factors, long-term prognosis, economic considerations, and ethical responsibility. Contemporary philosophy in conservative dentistry emphasizes preservation of the natural dentition whenever predictably feasible. However, preservation must not become dogma; it must be justified by biological, functional, and prognostic realism.

Pulpal diagnosis forms the biological starting point. A tooth diagnosed with reversible pulpitis may be managed conservatively with caries removal and indirect pulp therapy. In contrast, irreversible pulpitis or pulpal necrosis with apical periodontitis necessitates root canal therapy if the tooth is restorable. Diagnosis must be established through vitality testing, percussion, palpation, radiographic interpretation, and clinical correlation rather than radiographic appearance alone. A periapical radiolucency does not automatically mandate extraction; it often resolves following adequate chemomechanical debridement and obturation. Conversely, a tooth with necrosis but extensive vertical root fracture is non-salvageable despite correct pulpal diagnosis. Restorability is the structural determinant that frequently governs the final decision. A tooth may be endodontically treatable yet prosthodontically hopeless. Ferrule effect, remaining coronal dentin height, periodontal attachment levels, crown-root ratio, and presence of cracks must be evaluated before initiating treatment. Initiating endodontic therapy in a tooth lacking adequate ferrule or with subgingival caries extending beyond surgical correction exposes both patient and clinician to predictable failure. Restorability must therefore be assessed before, not after, root canal therapy. Prognosis depends on both biological and technical variables. Primary root canal therapy performed under proper aseptic isolation with thorough cleaning, shaping, and obturation demonstrates high long-term survival rates. Retreatment cases, however, require evaluation of cause of failure—missed canals, inadequate obturation, coronal leakage, or persistent infection. If retreatment can predictably eliminate etiologic factors, preservation remains rational. If anatomical complexities, ledging, perforation, or fractured instruments compromise outcome beyond recovery, extraction may be biologically more prudent.

Periodontal status significantly modifies prognosis. A tooth with isolated endodontic pathology but intact periodontal support typically responds favorably. However, combined endo-perio lesions require differentiation between primary endodontic lesions with secondary periodontal involvement and primary periodontal lesions with secondary pulpal involvement. Advanced horizontal bone loss with Grade III mobility significantly reduces long-term survival, even if endodontic treatment is technically successful. Implant considerations must be incorporated but not used as default justification for extraction. Implant survival rates are high, yet implants are not immune to complications such as peri-implant mucositis and peri-implantitis. Extraction followed by implant placement is a surgical procedure with systemic and local risk implications. Moreover, the long-term survival of well-treated natural teeth often equals or exceeds that of implants when maintenance is adequate. Therefore, extraction should be based on non-restorability or poor prognosis rather than perceived superiority of implant therapy.

Patient-centered considerations further influence decision-making. Systemic conditions such as uncontrolled diabetes, immunosuppression, or bisphosphonate therapy may alter surgical risk profiles. Financial capacity, compliance with maintenance, aesthetic expectations, and time constraints must be transparently discussed. Ethical communication requires explaining alternative options, success probabilities, and risks.

Medico-legally, documentation must demonstrate that restorability assessment preceded endodontic initiation, that alternatives including extraction and implant were discussed, and that informed consent was obtained. Initiating endodontic therapy on a non-restorable tooth without documentation exposes the practitioner to claims of unnecessary treatment.

Integrated Clinical Decision Table: Endodontic vs Extraction:

Clinical Parameter	Favor Endodontic Therapy	Favor Extraction	Clinical Insight
Pulpal Status	Irreversible pulpitis or necrosis without fracture	Vertical root fracture	Fracture lines dictate prognosis
Restorability	Adequate ferrule ≥2 mm,	Subgingival caries	Assess restorability

	manageable caries	beyond surgical correction	before RCT
Periodontal Support	Probing ≤5 mm, minimal mobility	Severe attachment loss, Grade III mobility	Periodontal stability predicts longevity
Crown-Root Ratio	Favorable ratio after restoration	Poor ratio even after crown lengthening	Structural biomechanics matter
Retreatment Feasibility	Missed canal identifiable and accessible	Perforation non-repairable, severe resorption	Cause of failure determines salvage
Patient Factors	Good oral hygiene, compliance	Poor compliance, unwilling to maintain	Maintenance influences survival
Implant Suitability	Contraindicated surgery or high risk	Adequate bone, systemic fitness	Compare biological cost
Strategic Value	Key abutment in fixed prosthesis	Non-strategic tooth	Consider overall rehabilitation plan

Clinical Illustration

A 38-year-old patient presents with symptomatic irreversible pulpitis in a mandibular first molar. Clinical examination reveals sufficient coronal tooth structure with 3 mm ferrule potential after crown placement. Periodontal probing shows 3–4 mm pockets without mobility. Radiograph reveals no vertical fracture. Decision pathway favors primary root canal therapy followed by full-coverage restoration. In contrast, a 55-year-old patient presents with necrotic pulp in a maxillary premolar with deep subgingival caries extending to the crestal bone and Grade II mobility. Even though endodontic treatment is technically possible, restorability and periodontal prognosis are compromised. Extraction with implant replacement becomes the rational decision.

```
Initial Assessment
 |
 ├── Confirm pulpal diagnosis
 |    |
 |    ├── Reversible pulpitis?
 |    |     └── Conservative restorative management
 |    |
 |    └── Irreversible pulpitis / Necrosis?
 |          |
 |          ├── Assess restorability
 |          |     |
 |          |     ├── Restorable?
 |          |     |     |
 |          |     |     ├── Evaluate periodontal status
 |          |     |     |     |
 |          |     |     |     ├── Adequate support?
 |          |     |     |     |     └── Root canal therapy
 |          |     |     |     |
 |          |     |     |     └── Poor support?
 |          |     |     |           └── Consider extraction
 |          |     |     |
 |          |     |     └── Non-restorable?
 |          |     |           └── Extraction
 |          |     |
 |          |     └── Retreatment case?
 |          |           |
 |          |           ├── Cause identifiable & correctable?
 |          |           |     └── Nonsurgical or surgical retreatment
 |          |           |
 |          |           └── Non-correctable defect?
 |          |                 └── Extraction
 |
 └── Post-extraction planning
      |
      ├── Adequate bone & systemic health?
      |     └── Implant placement
      |
      └── Alternative prosthetic options
            └── Fixed or removable prosthesis
```

Restorative Material Selection

Dr. P.Bravin Paul
Department : M.D.S (Orthodontics & Dentofacial Orthopedics)
Clinic Name: Dr. Paul's Dental & Orthodontic Care
Madurai, Tamil Nadu, Pincode : 625706, India

Clinical choices among composites, ceramics, metals, and biomaterials.

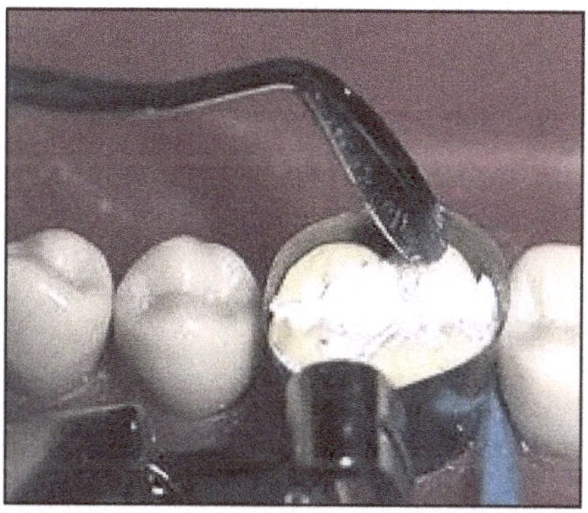

Restorative material selection is not a purely technical decision but a biologically informed, biomechanically calculated, and patient-centered judgment. The clinician must weigh esthetic demands, occlusal forces, remaining tooth structure, caries risk, moisture control feasibility, longevity expectations, cost considerations, and the patient's systemic profile before selecting among direct composites, indirect ceramics, metallic restorations, or contemporary bioactive materials. The evolution of adhesive dentistry has expanded conservative treatment options; however, material choice must align with functional risk and long-term prognosis rather than aesthetic preference alone.

Composite resins have transformed minimally invasive dentistry by allowing adhesive, tooth-colored restorations that preserve enamel and dentin. Their ability to bond micromechanically and chemically to tooth structure supports conservative cavity preparation. However, polymerization shrinkage stress, technique sensitivity, and wear under heavy occlusal loads remain concerns. In posterior stress-bearing regions, the operator must evaluate cusp thickness and consider cusp coverage when indicated. A small Class I lesion in a low caries-risk patient is an ideal indication; a large MOD cavity in a bruxer may require reinforcement or indirect restoration instead.

Ceramic materials offer superior esthetics, color stability, and compressive strength. Lithium disilicate and zirconia-based systems allow full-coverage crowns, onlays, and veneers with excellent longevity when bonded or conventionally cemented appropriately. However, ceramics are brittle and require adequate thickness and ferrule. Occlusal clearance, preparation geometry, and parafunctional habits must be evaluated. A thin ceramic restoration placed without sufficient reduction may fracture prematurely despite ideal bonding.

Metallic restorations, including high noble and base metal alloys, provide exceptional strength and longevity, especially in posterior load-bearing areas. Cast gold restorations remain one of the most durable options, exhibiting minimal wear to opposing dentition and excellent marginal adaptation. Their declining use is primarily due to esthetic demands rather than functional limitations. In high occlusal stress patients or when isolation is compromised, metallic restorations may outperform adhesive alternatives.

Contemporary biomaterials, including resin-modified glass ionomers and bioactive restorative systems, provide fluoride release and chemical bonding to tooth structure. They are particularly valuable in high caries-risk patients, pediatric dentistry, geriatric populations, and cases where moisture control is difficult. However, their lower wear resistance limits use in large stress-bearing restorations.

Material selection must therefore align with a structured evaluation: assess lesion size, load distribution, enamel availability for bonding, esthetic zone involvement, and patient-specific risk. Overuse of highly aesthetic materials in high-stress zones or reliance on metallic restorations in highly visible areas without patient consent reflects incomplete decision-making. Ethical practice requires informed discussion of alternatives, expected longevity, maintenance needs, and potential complications.

Medico-legally, documentation should justify material selection based on clinical findings. Failure of a restoration may not constitute negligence if selection was rational and consent documented. Conversely, choosing an inadequate material for a high-load situation without documentation may be defensible neither biologically nor legally.

Interactive Example-Based Comparative Table: Composition–Function–Clinical Illustration

Material Category	Composition	Primary Functional Properties	Ideal Clinical Indication	Clinical Illustration	Key Limitation
Direct Composite Resin	Resin matrix (Bis-GMA/UDMA), filler particles (silica, zirconia), coupling agent	Adhesive bonding, esthetics, moderate strength	Small–moderate anterior or posterior restorations	28-year-old with small Class II lesion restored conservatively with bonded composite	Polymerization shrinkage, wear in bruxers
Bulk-Fill Composite	Modified resin matrix with	Deeper curing, reduced shrinkage	Posterior restorations	35-year-old molar cavity	Technique sensitive

	stress-relieving monomers	stress	requiring efficient placement	restored in 4 mm increments	curing
Lithium Disilicate Ceramic	Glass-ceramic with lithium disilicate crystals	High esthetics, good flexural strength	Anterior crowns, onlays, veneers	Fractured incisor restored with bonded ceramic crown	Requires sufficient thickness
Zirconia	Polycrystalline ceramic (yttria-stabilized zirconium oxide)	High fracture toughness, strength	Posterior crowns, bridges	Bruxer patient receives monolithic zirconia crown	Less translucency than glass ceramics
Cast Gold Alloy	High noble alloy (gold, platinum, palladium)	Excellent durability, marginal integrity	Posterior inlay/onlay in high-load case	50-year-old with heavy occlusion restored with gold onlay	Poor esthetics
Amalgam (where still	Silver-tin alloy with mercury	High compressive strength,	Large posterior restora	Deep molar restoration in	Esthetic and environmenta

used)		moisture tolerance	tions with limited isolation	limited moisture control	l concerns
Resin-Modified Glass Ionomer	Fluoroaluminosilicate glass + resin components	Fluoride release, chemical bonding	Cervical lesions, pediatric cases	Root caries restored in elderly xerostomic patient	Lower wear resistance
Bioactive Restorative Material	Calcium-phosphate or ion-releasing matrix	Remineralization support	High caries-risk patients	Young patient with recurrent caries risk receives bioactive restoration	Limited long-term evidence

Clinical Decision Illustration

Consider a 40-year-old patient presenting with a fractured mesiobuccal cusp of a mandibular molar. Remaining tooth structure is thin, and occlusal load is high. A direct composite may temporarily restore form but risks cusp flexure and fracture. An indirect lithium disilicate onlay bonded with adhesive cement provides cusp coverage and reinforcement. If the patient demonstrates severe bruxism, monolithic zirconia may be more fracture-resistant.

In contrast, a 22-year-old patient with a small proximal lesion in a premolar with intact cusps is best managed with a conservative composite restoration, preserving enamel and avoiding aggressive preparation.

Conceptual Integration

Material selection should not follow aesthetic trends or habitual preference but structured evaluation of biomechanics, biology, and patient context. The clinician must think beyond immediate restoration placement and envision functional longevity, periodontal harmony, and maintenance feasibility. Conservative dentistry does not mean weak dentistry; strength does not require overtreatment. The optimal restorative material is the one that harmonizes mechanical demand with biological preservation and patient-centered expectations.

Prosthodontic Treatment Decisions

Dr. Rahul Puthenkandathil
Lecturer
Nitte (deemed to be University),
AB Shetty Memorial institute of Dental Sciences,
Department of Prosthodontics and Crown and Bridge.
Mangaluru - 575018 Karnataka, India

Fixed, removable, implant-supported prostheses—case selection and outcomes.

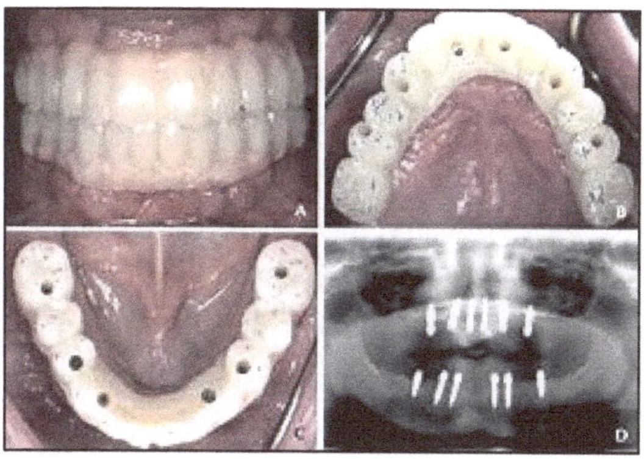

Prosthodontic treatment planning represents a synthesis of biological evaluation, biomechanical forecasting, aesthetic design, and patient-centered dialogue. The decision between fixed dental prostheses, removable prostheses, and implant-supported restorations is not merely restorative—it is reconstructive. It demands careful assessment of residual dentition, periodontal stability, bone volume, occlusal scheme, systemic health, patient dexterity, financial capacity, and long-term maintenance feasibility. The objective is not simply replacement of missing teeth but restoration of function, phonetics, comfort, and psychosocial well-being while minimizing biological cost.

Fixed dental prostheses (FDPs), including single crowns and fixed partial dentures, remain foundational in partially edentulous rehabilitation.

Their success depends heavily on abutment tooth health, periodontal support, crown-root ratio, and occlusal loading patterns. The preparation of abutment teeth involves irreversible removal of tooth structure; therefore, biological cost must be justified by expected longevity. A three-unit bridge replacing a missing premolar may function predictably when adjacent teeth are heavily restored and periodontally sound. However, preparing intact virgin teeth solely to avoid implant placement may be biologically excessive. Long-term outcomes of FDPs correlate with marginal integrity, connector design, occlusal harmony, and patient hygiene compliance. Secondary caries and periodontal breakdown around abutments are primary causes of failure.

Removable partial dentures (RPDs) and complete dentures continue to play an essential role, particularly in medically compromised, elderly, or financially constrained patients. Removable prostheses provide reversible, conservative treatment with minimal tooth preparation. However, their success depends on meticulous design principles—appropriate clasp assembly, support, bracing, indirect retention, and major connector rigidity. Poorly designed RPDs can accelerate periodontal deterioration and caries development in abutment teeth. Complete dentures require careful consideration of residual ridge morphology, neuromuscular coordination, salivary flow, and patient adaptability. Psychological acceptance is as critical as technical fabrication. While removable options may not replicate natural dentition fully, they remain biologically conservative and adaptable solutions in appropriate cases.

Implant-supported prostheses have transformed modern prosthodontics by eliminating the need to prepare adjacent teeth and by preserving alveolar bone through functional stimulation. Single-tooth implants, implant-supported fixed bridges, and implant-retained overdentures provide enhanced stability and patient satisfaction. Nevertheless, implant therapy is a surgical intervention and must be evaluated within systemic and local risk frameworks. Bone volume and quality, soft tissue biotype, occlusal forces, parafunctional habits, smoking status, glycemic control, and patient compliance significantly influence outcomes. Although survival rates are high, complications such as peri-implant mucositis, peri-implantitis, screw loosening, and prosthetic fracture are documented. Therefore, implant therapy should not be positioned as universally superior but as one modality within a comprehensive decision matrix.

Case selection must begin with a comprehensive diagnostic phase: full-mouth periodontal evaluation, occlusal analysis, radiographic imaging, assessment of vertical dimension, interarch space measurement, and evaluation of esthetic parameters. Strategic importance of remaining teeth must be determined. A patient with a single missing molar and intact adjacent teeth may benefit from an implant rather than a fixed bridge. Conversely, a patient with multiple failing teeth and reduced periodontal support may be better managed with a removable prosthesis rather than multiple implants with questionable prognosis.

Outcomes assessment should consider both survival and success. Survival refers to the prosthesis remaining in situ; success implies absence of biological or mechanical complications. Fixed prostheses often demonstrate high survival but may require maintenance such as recementation or repair. Removable prostheses may require periodic relining due to ridge resorption. Implant-supported prostheses show high survival but demand strict maintenance protocols to prevent peri-implant disease. Long-term maintenance is therefore integral to treatment planning, not an afterthought.

Occlusion plays a pivotal role in prosthodontic longevity. Uncontrolled occlusal forces can jeopardize both natural abutments and implants. Implant-supported restorations lack periodontal ligament proprioception, altering force distribution. Therefore, occlusal schemes must be carefully designed to reduce overload, particularly in bruxers.

Patient expectations must be explored thoroughly. Some patients prioritize fixed solutions for psychological comfort; others may accept removable options for economic or surgical reasons. Informed consent should include discussion of advantages, limitations, maintenance requirements, longevity expectations, and potential complications. Ethical prosthodontics balances patient preference with biological prudence.

Medico-legally, documentation of diagnostic findings, alternative options presented, risk assessment, and patient consent is essential. Failure of a prosthesis does not equate to negligence if case selection and communication were appropriate. However, placing implants in uncontrolled diabetic patients without medical consultation or preparing periodontally compromised abutments without stabilization may constitute deviation from accepted standards of care.

Ultimately, prosthodontic treatment decisions should be guided by a hierarchy of preservation: maintain healthy natural teeth whenever possible, replace missing structures conservatively, and select implant therapy when it offers clear biomechanical and biological advantage. The best prosthesis is not defined by material or technology but by its harmony with the patient's biology, function, and long-term maintainability.

Integrated Comparative Decision Matrix with Clinical Scenarios:

Clinical Scenario	Fixed Dental Prosthesis (FDP)	Removable Prosthesis	Implant-Supported Prosthesis	Preferred Option & Rationale	Long-Term Consideration
Single missing posterior tooth; adjacent teeth intact	Requires preparation of healthy abutments	Not ideal for single-tooth replacement	Preserves adjacent teeth; high function	Implant-supported crown – conservative to adjacent teeth	Requires surgical suitability and maintenance
Single	Logical	Possible	Implant	FDP –	Monito

missing tooth; adjacent teeth heavily restored	to use as abutments	but unnecessary bulk	possible but higher cost	utilizes already restored teeth	r abutment caries risk
Multiple missing posterior teeth; distal extension	Limited without posterior abutment	RPD feasible and conservative	Multiple implants possible	RPD or implant-supported prosthesis depending on finances and bone	Maintenance critical to prevent abutment overload
Completely edentulous maxilla	Not applicable	Complete denture	Implant-supported overdenture or full-arch fixed	Implant overdenture if bone adequate; otherwise complete denture	Ridge resorption management
Periodontally compromised remaining teeth	Risk of abutment failure	Removable option safer	Implants may be compromised in poor hygiene	Removable prosthesis until periodontal	Compliance determines prognosis

				stability achieved	
Bruxism patient	Risk of connector fracture	May cause tissue trauma	Implant restoration risk of overload	Carefully designed FDP or reinforced implant with occlusal guard	Occlusal protection mandatory
Medically compromised patient (uncontrolled diabetes)	Possible if teeth stable	Conservative and reversible	Surgical risk elevated	Removable prosthesis initially	Reassess after medical stabilization
Limited interarch space	Preparation may weaken abutments	Acrylic design adaptable	Implant prosthesis requires precise planning	Case-dependent	Evaluate vertical dimension carefully

Occlusion and Temporomandibular Disorders

Dr. Manaswi Tripathi Mishra
MDS (Oral & Maxillofacial Surgery)
Assistant Professor
S.M.S Medical college & Attached Hospital,Jaipur (Rajasthan)

Diagnosis-based management decisions and risk–benefit analysis.

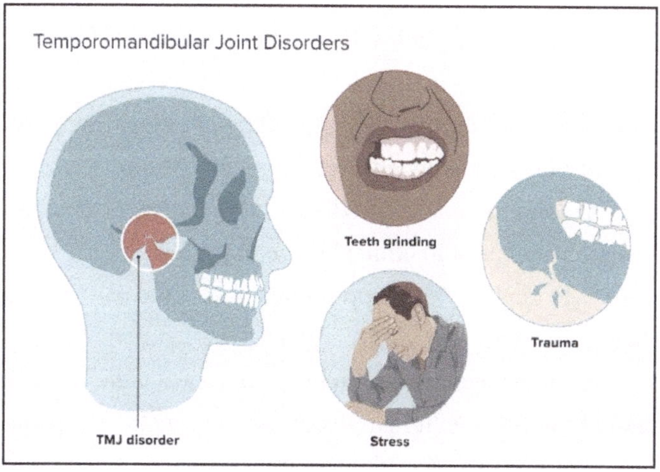

Occlusion and temporomandibular disorders (TMDs) occupy one of the most debated intersections in dentistry, where biomechanical theory, neuromuscular physiology, and psychosocial variables converge. Historically, occlusion was considered a primary etiological factor in TMD; contemporary evidence suggests a multifactorial model in which occlusal discrepancies may act as modifying rather than sole causative factors. Therefore, management must be diagnosis-driven rather than mechanically reactive. The clinician's responsibility is to differentiate between adaptive occlusal variations and pathologic dysfunction requiring intervention.

TMD encompasses a spectrum of conditions involving the temporomandibular joint (TMJ), masticatory muscles, or associated structures. According to the diagnostic framework proposed by the Diagnostic Criteria for Temporomandibular Disorders, TMD can be broadly categorized into muscle disorders (myalgia, myofascial pain), joint disorders (disc displacement with or without reduction), degenerative joint disease, and headache attributed to TMD. Each category requires distinct clinical reasoning; blanket occlusal adjustment is neither evidence-based nor ethically defensible.

Occlusal evaluation must include assessment of intercuspal position, centric relation stability, occlusal interferences, wear facets, fremitus, mobility, and parafunctional signs. However, the presence of an occlusal discrepancy does not automatically indicate pathology. Many individuals exhibit occlusal interferences yet remain asymptomatic due to neuromuscular adaptation. The distinction between adaptation and decompensation is central to clinical decision-making.

Diagnosis begins with comprehensive history taking: pain characteristics, onset, duration, aggravating factors, joint sounds, limitation of movement, headaches, psychosocial stressors, and parafunctional habits. Clinical examination includes palpation of masticatory muscles, joint auscultation, measurement of mandibular range of motion, and evaluation of deviation patterns. Imaging may be indicated in specific scenarios; panoramic radiography for gross structural evaluation and advanced imaging when degenerative changes or disc pathology are suspected.

Management decisions must be proportional to diagnosis severity. In myogenous TMD without structural joint pathology, conservative therapy—education, reassurance, behavioral modification, physiotherapy, and occlusal splints—is often sufficient. Occlusal splints redistribute occlusal forces, reduce muscle hyperactivity, and protect dentition from parafunctional wear. However, splints are adjunctive, not curative, and must be monitored for occlusal changes.

Irreversible occlusal adjustments or full-mouth rehabilitation should not be first-line therapy for pain-dominant TMD. The risk–benefit ratio must be carefully weighed. Permanent occlusal alteration carries risks of postoperative sensitivity, altered vertical dimension, pulpal complications, and patient dissatisfaction if symptoms persist. Evidence indicates that conservative reversible therapy achieves comparable outcomes in many cases, emphasizing the principle of minimal intervention.

Disc displacement with reduction, characterized by clicking without pain, may not require active intervention beyond monitoring. Disc displacement without reduction accompanied by limited opening may necessitate anti-inflammatory management, physiotherapy, or referral to a specialist. Degenerative joint disease may require pharmacologic therapy, occlusal stabilization, or multidisciplinary management involving rheumatology or pain specialists. Psychosocial factors play a substantial role. Stress, anxiety, and sleep disorders contribute significantly to parafunctional activity such as bruxism. Therefore, TMD management may extend beyond occlusal correction to include cognitive behavioral strategies and interdisciplinary referral.

Risk–benefit analysis in occlusal intervention should consider:

Biological Risk: irreversible tooth structure removal, pulp damage, periodontal trauma.

Functional Risk: altered occlusal scheme causing new dysfunction. Psychological Risk: unmet expectations or persistence of symptoms. Benefit: symptom relief, improved function, prevention of further structural damage. For example, a patient presenting with generalized occlusal wear but no pain may not require extensive rehabilitation if function is stable. Conversely, severe bruxism causing fractures and muscle pain may benefit from protective splint therapy before definitive restorative planning. Medico-legally, occlusion-related litigation often arises from irreversible occlusal adjustments performed without documented diagnosis. Proper documentation should include baseline occlusal records, mounted diagnostic casts when indicated, informed consent outlining uncertainty of symptom resolution, and documentation of conservative options offered. The clinician must avoid promising symptom elimination solely through occlusal correction.

In restorative cases involving full-mouth rehabilitation, occlusal planning becomes preventive rather than therapeutic. Establishing stable centric contacts, appropriate anterior guidance, and posterior disclusion reduces overload risk. Implant restorations require particular caution, as implants lack periodontal ligament proprioception and are more susceptible to overload-induced complications.

Ultimately, occlusion should be viewed as a dynamic functional relationship rather than a static ideal. The goal is not to achieve theoretical perfection but to maintain comfortable function within physiologic tolerance. Diagnosis-based management prioritizes reversible therapy, patient education, and cautious progression to irreversible procedures only when justified by persistent dysfunction and comprehensive evaluation.

Diagnosis-Based Management and Risk–Benefit Analysis (Integrated Table):

Diagnostic Category	Key Clinical Features	Occlusal Findings	Primary Management Approach	Reversibility Level	Risk–Benefit Consideration	Clinical Decision Insight
Myalgia / Myofascial Pain	Diffuse muscle tenderness, fatigue, morning stiffne	May have wear facets, but occlusion often adaptive	Patient education, physiotherapy, behavioral therapy, occlusal splint	Reversible	Low biological risk; high symptom relief potential	Avoid irreversible occlusal adjustment initially

	ss					
Parafunction (Bruxism-related overload)	Tooth wear, fractures, muscle hypertrophy	Flattened cusps, fremitus	Night guard (stabilization splint), stress management	Reversible	Protects dentition; minimal harm	Splint before definitive restorative rehabilitation
Disc Displacement with Reduction	Joint clicking, normal opening	Usually incidental occlusal variation	Observation, reassurance, monitoring	Reversible	Intervention may be unnecessary	Treat symptoms, not sounds
Disc Displacement without Reduction	Limited opening, deviation, pain	Not primarily occlusion-driven	Anti-inflammatory therapy, physiotherapy, splint	Reversible	Early conservative care improves prognosis	Avoid aggressive occlusal alteration
Degenerative Joint Disease	Crepitus, radiographic changes, chronic pain	Secondary occlusal changes possible	Pharmacologic therapy, stabilization splint, referral if	Mostly reversible (except structural damage)	Surgery rarely first-line	Multidisciplinary management often required

			severe			
Occlusal Instability after Restorative Work	Sudden discomfort after new crown/ bridge	High spot or interference	Selective occlusal adjustment (minor)	Partially irreversible	Benefit outweighs minimal enamel adjustment	Confirm with articulating paper and shimstock
Severe Malocclusion with Functional Impairment	Recurrent trauma, mobility, fracture	Unstable centric relation–centric occlusion discrepancy	Comprehensive occlusal rehabilitation	Irreversible	High cost and biological risk; indicated only if dysfunction confirmed	Mount casts and document baseline records
Asymptomatic Occlusal Discrepancy	No pain or dysfunction	Minor interference	No treatment	—	Risk of overtreatment exceeds benefit	Observation preferred

Surgical Decision-Making

Dr. Anish Nelson
Lecturer, Nitte (Deemed to be university), Ab Shetty memorial Institute of Dental Sciences (ABSMIDS), Department of Oral and Maxillofacial surgery, Mangalore, India

Extractions, implants, grafts, soft tissue surgery, and minimally invasive approaches.

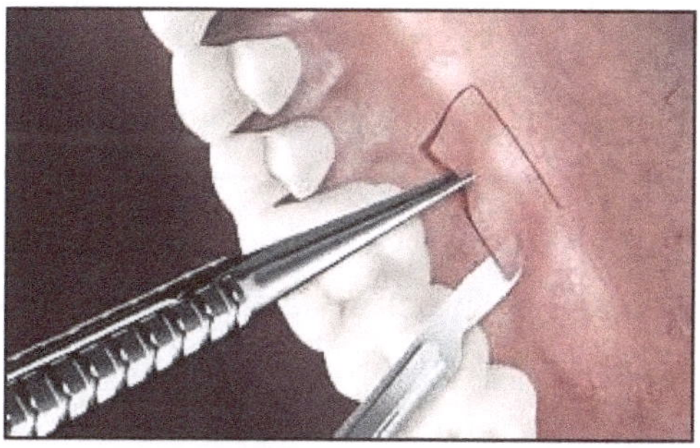

Surgical decision-making in dentistry requires integration of diagnosis, anatomical assessment, systemic risk evaluation, patient-centered expectations, technical feasibility, and long-term biological consequences. The clinician must weigh not only whether a procedure can be performed, but whether it should be performed. Ethical and medico-legal defensibility depends on proportionality—intervention should correspond to disease severity and prognosis. Surgical treatment is justified when conservative measures are inadequate, prognosis is compromised, or structural rehabilitation necessitates intervention.

Surgical planning begins with comprehensive assessment: medical history, radiographic imaging, periodontal evaluation, occlusal analysis, and soft tissue examination. Systemic conditions such as uncontrolled diabetes, bleeding disorders, immunosuppression, osteoporosis therapy (particularly bisphosphonates), and cardiovascular disease significantly influence surgical risk. Failure to identify or appropriately manage systemic risk factors constitutes a breach of standard care.

1. Extractions: Indications, Technique, and Risk Assessment

Tooth extraction is indicated when a tooth is non-restorable due to extensive caries, vertical root fracture, severe periodontal destruction, or persistent infection unresponsive to treatment. However, extraction must never be the default alternative to technically demanding restorative therapy. The decision requires confirmation of hopeless prognosis, documentation of restorability assessment, and discussion of replacement options.

Surgically, atraumatic technique is paramount. Preoperative radiographs assess root morphology, proximity to anatomical structures such as the inferior alveolar nerve or maxillary sinus, and presence of pathology. Sectioning multirooted teeth reduces alveolar trauma. Excessive force increases risk of cortical plate fracture or nerve injury.

Medico-legal case example:

A patient underwent mandibular third molar extraction without documented radiographic evaluation. Postoperative paresthesia developed due to inferior alveolar nerve injury. Lack of documented risk disclosure and imaging constituted negligence. Proper documentation of nerve proximity and informed consent would have strengthened legal defensibility.

2. Implant Placement: Indications and Surgical Phases

Implant surgery must be diagnosis-driven, not marketing-driven. Indications include single-tooth replacement without compromising adjacent teeth, support for distal extension cases, and retention of complete dentures. Contraindications include uncontrolled systemic disease, inadequate bone without augmentation feasibility, active periodontal infection, or poor compliance.

Surgical planning includes CBCT assessment for bone volume, proximity to anatomical landmarks, and prosthetically driven positioning.

The sequence includes flap design or flapless approach (when appropriate), osteotomy preparation with controlled irrigation to prevent thermal necrosis, implant placement with primary stability, and suturing. Healing may be submerged or transmucosal depending on stability and protocol. Risk factors include peri-implantitis, nerve injury, sinus perforation, and implant failure due to overload. Implants lack periodontal ligament proprioception; occlusal overload is a recognized cause of marginal bone loss.

Medico-legal case example:

An implant was placed in a heavy smoker with uncontrolled diabetes without medical consultation. Early implant failure occurred. Absence of risk documentation and failure to advise on smoking cessation led to litigation for inappropriate case selection.

3. Bone Grafting and Regenerative Surgery

Bone grafting may be indicated for ridge augmentation, sinus lift procedures, or periodontal regeneration. Materials include autografts, allografts, xenografts, and alloplasts. Selection depends on defect morphology, volume required, and systemic compatibility.

In sinus augmentation, Schneiderian membrane integrity must be preserved. Perforation management includes membrane repair and staged healing. Excessive graft placement can lead to sinus complications.

Regenerative periodontal surgery requires careful case selection. Three-wall intrabony defects respond better to guided tissue regeneration than one-wall defects. Smoking significantly reduces regenerative outcomes.

Medico-legal case example:

A sinus lift procedure was performed without preoperative sinus evaluation. Postoperative sinusitis developed. Failure to obtain appropriate imaging and medical consultation constituted deviation from accepted protocol.

4. Soft Tissue Surgery

Soft tissue procedures include crown lengthening, frenectomy, gingivectomy, and mucogingival surgery. Indications must be biologically justified. Crown lengthening should consider biologic width and future restorative margins. Excessive removal of supporting bone to facilitate restoration may compromise long-term periodontal stability.

Mucogingival grafts are indicated for progressive recession with sensitivity or aesthetic concern. However, asymptomatic recession without progression may not require surgery.

Medico-legal case example:

Aesthetic crown lengthening was performed without discussion of potential root sensitivity and altered gingival contour. Patient dissatisfaction resulted in claim of inadequate consent. Proper preoperative photographic documentation and consent would have mitigated risk.

5. Minimally Invasive Surgical Approaches

Modern dentistry emphasizes minimally invasive surgery—preservation of bone and soft tissue through flapless implant placement (when indicated), microsurgical techniques, piezosurgery, and atraumatic extraction methods. These approaches reduce morbidity and accelerate healing but require advanced training and case selection.

Minimally invasive techniques are not universally applicable. Limited visibility in complex anatomy may increase risk if improperly selected.

Integrated Surgical Decision Table

Surgical Procedure	Primary Indication	Contraindication	Key Risk	Preventive Strategy	Medico-Legal Safeguard
Extraction	Non-restorab	Salvageable with	Nerve injury	Preoperative	Document

	le tooth	predictable therapy		imaging	prognosis discussion
Implant Placement	Missing tooth, adequate bone	Uncontrolled systemic disease	Peri-implantitis	Risk factor modification	Informed consent detailing alternatives
Sinus Lift	Insufficient posterior maxillary bone	Active sinus pathology	Membrane perforation	CBCT planning	ENT consultation documentation
Ridge Augmentation	Horizontal deficiency	Poor healing potential	Graft failure	Smoking cessation	Material disclosure consent
Crown Lengthening	Subgingival margin, altered passive eruption	Short root length	Attachment loss	Biological width preservation	Photographic documentation
Soft Tissue Graft	Progressive recession	Stable asymptomatic recession	Graft necrosis	Vascular bed preparation	Explain aesthetic variability

Risk–Benefit Framework in Surgical Decision-Making

Consideration	Low-Risk Conservative	Moderate Surgical	Advanced Surgical

Biological Cost	Minimal	Moderate	High
Reversibility	High	Limited	Irreversible
Patient Morbidity	Minimal	Moderate swelling/pain	Significant
Justification Threshold	Low	Moderate	High

Ethical and Legal Principles

Surgical dentistry requires:

Comprehensive diagnosis before intervention. Clear documentation of alternatives. Informed consent explaining risks, benefits, and uncertainties. Postoperative monitoring and complication management.

Failure to diagnose is more litigated than failure of surgery. Proper records, imaging, risk assessment, and documented communication form the core of medico-legal protection.

Orthodontic and Interdisciplinary Decisions

Dr. Ramandeep Kaur
Designation: Assistant Professor
College currently affiliated with: Rajshree medical College,
Bareilly, Uttar Pradesh

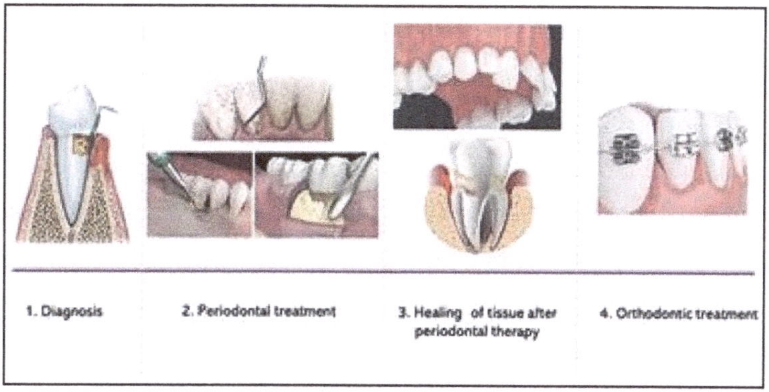

Clinical decision-making in dentistry is rarely confined to a single specialty. In contemporary practice, orthodontics is no longer viewed as an isolated tooth-alignment discipline but as a biological, functional, and esthetic foundation for comprehensive rehabilitation. Orthodontic decisions influence periodontal stability, prosthodontic longevity, implant positioning, occlusal harmony, and even facial esthetics.

For the clinician, the essential questions are:

- **When should orthodontic intervention begin?**
- **When should a patient be referred?**
- **How should orthodontic treatment be sequenced with periodontal, restorative, prosthetic, or implant therapy?**

Orthodontic and interdisciplinary planning is not merely about aligning teeth; it is about **creating ideal biological conditions for long-term stability and restorative predictability**. This chapter explores the principles of timing, referral protocols, interdisciplinary integration, and practical decision-making frameworks in comprehensive dental care.

1. Biological Foundations of Orthodontic Decision-Making

Orthodontic movement is fundamentally a biologic response involving:

- Periodontal ligament remodeling
- Alveolar bone resorption and apposition
- Soft tissue adaptation
- Neuromuscular equilibrium

Understanding this biology is essential before integrating orthodontics into interdisciplinary planning.

1.1 Periodontal Considerations

Orthodontic movement is safe in a **healthy periodontium**. However:

- Active periodontal disease increases risk of attachment loss.
- Reduced bone height alters center of resistance.
- Excessive forces may lead to further bone loss.

Thus, **periodontal stabilization precedes orthodontic therapy** in compromised patients.

1.2 Growth Considerations

In growing patients:

- Skeletal discrepancies can be modified.
- Timing is critical for Class II and Class III correction.
- Functional appliances rely on pubertal growth spurt.

In adults:

- Orthodontics is primarily dentoalveolar.
- Combined surgical approaches may be needed.

2. Timing of Orthodontic Intervention

Orthodontic timing is broadly categorized into:

- **Preventive phase**
- **Interceptive phase**
- **Comprehensive phase**
- **Adjunctive orthodontics in adults**

2.1 Preventive Orthodontics

Includes:

- Space maintenance
- Early extraction guidance
- Habit interception

Goal: Prevent development of malocclusion.

2.2 Interceptive Orthodontics (Mixed Dentition Phase)

Age: 7–11 years

Indications:

- Crossbite correction
- Severe crowding
- Skeletal Class II with mandibular retrusion
- Developing Class III patterns

Early intervention reduces complexity of later treatment.

2.3 Comprehensive Orthodontics (Adolescent Phase)

Age: 11–14 years

Optimal for:

- Full fixed appliance therapy
- Growth modification during peak pubertal growth

2.4 Adult Orthodontics

Indications:

- Pre-prosthetic space redistribution
- Implant site development
- Periodontally compromised cases
- Orthognathic surgery preparation

Adult orthodontics requires interdisciplinary collaboration.

3. Referral Protocols: When and Why?

General dentists play a pivotal role in early detection and referral.

3.1 Indications for Orthodontic Referral

- Skeletal discrepancies
- Severe crowding (>6 mm)
- Impacted teeth
- Midline deviations

- Traumatic deep bite
- Open bite
- Pre-prosthetic space management
- Periodontally compromised migration

3.2 Red Flags for Immediate Referral

- Asymmetric mandibular growth
- Progressive anterior crossbite
- Impacted canines
- Severe skeletal Class III in early childhood

Timely referral prevents irreversible complications.

4. Interdisciplinary Orthodontic–Periodontal Planning

Periodontal health and orthodontics share a delicate relationship.

4.1 Sequence of Care

1. Phase I periodontal therapy
2. Re-evaluation
3. Orthodontic treatment
4. Periodontal recontouring or regenerative procedures
5. Maintenance phase

4.2 Orthodontics in Periodontally Compromised Patients

Benefits include:

- Uprighting tilted molars
- Closing pathological migration spaces
- Improving oral hygiene access

However:

- Forces must be lighter.
- Movement must remain within alveolar housing.
- Frequent periodontal monitoring is mandatory.

4.3 Forced Eruption (Orthodontic Extrusion)

Used for:

- Crown lengthening
- Fractured tooth management

- Improving ferrule effect before prosthetic restoration

5. Orthodontic–Prosthodontic Integration

Orthodontics often prepares the foundation for ideal prosthetic outcomes.

5.1 Pre-Prosthetic Orthodontics

Objectives:

- Redistribute space
- Correct axial inclinations
- Improve crown-root ratio
- Align occlusal plane

Example:

Before placing veneers, minor orthodontics may correct rotations and spacing to conserve tooth structure.

5.2 Implant Site Development

Orthodontics is essential for:

- Space opening for congenitally missing lateral incisors
- Root parallelism before implant placement
- Vertical site development

Improper spacing compromises implant positioning and esthetics.

5.3 Adult Multidisciplinary Rehabilitation

Cases may include:

- Orthodontics
- Periodontal surgery
- Implants
- Full mouth rehabilitation

Treatment sequencing is crucial.

6. Orthodontics and Endodontic Considerations

- Previously treated teeth can be moved.
- Periapical pathology must be resolved before movement.
- Root resorption risk increases in certain cases.

Endodontic clearance is recommended prior to orthodontic force application.

7. Orthodontics and Orthognathic Surgery

In severe skeletal discrepancies:

- Presurgical orthodontics aligns teeth.
- Surgical repositioning corrects skeletal base.
- Postsurgical orthodontics refines occlusion.

Clear communication between surgeon and orthodontist is mandatory.

8. Digital Workflow in Interdisciplinary Planning

Modern interdisciplinary planning involves:

- CBCT imaging
- Digital smile design
- Virtual orthodontic setups
- Guided implant surgery

Digital tools enhance precision in combined therapy.

9. Clinical Decision-Making Algorithm

A structured approach includes:

1. Chief complaint analysis
2. Skeletal vs dental diagnosis
3. Periodontal assessment
4. Growth evaluation
5. Esthetic assessment
6. Restorative prognosis
7. Sequencing plan
8. Interdisciplinary consultation

10. Case-Based Clinical Scenarios

Case 1: Adult with Pathologic Migration

Findings:

- Periodontal bone loss
- Flaring of anterior teeth
- Diastema formation

Management:

- Periodontal therapy
- Light orthodontic alignment
- Splinting if needed

Case 2: Missing Lateral Incisor

Decision:

- Space closure vs implant

Factors:

- Facial profile
- Smile line
- Gingival biotype
- Patient age

Case 3: Deep Bite with Prosthetic Wear

Management:

- Orthodontic intrusion
- Increase vertical dimension
- Prosthetic rehabilitation

11. Risk Assessment in Interdisciplinary Orthodontics

11.1 Root Resorption

Higher risk in:

- Prolonged treatment
- Heavy forces
- Previous trauma

11.2 Periodontal Breakdown

Risk in:

- Poor plaque control
- Smokers
- Uncontrolled diabetes

11.3 Relapse

Common in:

- Rotated teeth
- Spacing cases
- Open bite correction

Retention protocols are essential.

12. Retention in Interdisciplinary Cases

Retention must consider:

- Periodontal stability
- Prosthetic margins
- Implant restorations
- Occlusal scheme

Permanent bonded retainers are often indicated.

Clinical Tips for Orthodontic and Interdisciplinary Decision-Making

Clinical Scenario	Decision Principle	Timing	Interdisciplinary Coordination	Clinical Tip
Periodontally compromised anterior flaring	Stabilize periodontium first	Before orthodontics	Periodontist	Use light forces and frequent recalls
Congenitally missing lateral incisor	Space closure vs implant decision	During adolescence planning	Orthodontist + Prosthodontist	Maintain ideal root parallelism for implants
Impacted	Early	Age 9–11	Orthodontist	CBCT

canine	radiographic screening		+ Oral surgeon	for 3D localization
Deep bite with attrition	Orthodontic intrusion	Before prosthetic rehabilitation	Prosthodontist	Avoid increasing VDO without orthodontic planning
Tilted molar adjacent to edentulous space	Uprighting orthodontically	Before implant	Orthodontist	Uprighting improves periodontal health
Fractured tooth requiring ferrule	Forced eruption	Before crown	Periodontist	Maintain biologic width
Skeletal Class II adolescent	Growth modification	Pubertal growth spurt	Orthodontist	Monitor growth with CVMI staging
Adult full mouth rehab	Pre-prosthetic orthodontics	Before final prosthesis	Prosthodontist	Digital wax-up aids sequencing
Midline deviation	Identify skeletal vs dental	Early diagnosis	Orthodontist	Early correction

	cause			prevents asymmetry progression
Severe crowding in mixed dentition	Interceptive extraction planning	Age 8–10	Pediatric dentist	Preserve leeway space

13. Ethical and Communication Considerations

Interdisciplinary cases demand:

- Informed consent
- Clear explanation of sequencing
- Realistic outcome discussion
- Documentation of collaborative planning

Patient-centered decision-making remains paramount.

Managing Complications and Failures

Dr. Pallavi
Senior resident,
Department of conservative dentistry and endodontics,
Swami devi dayal dental college and hospital,panchkula

Diagnosis of failures, revision strategies, and medico-legal considerations.

Complications and failures are inherent to clinical practice, not reflections of incompetence but of biological variability, material limitations, and patient-specific risk factors. The distinction between a complication and negligence lies not in the occurrence of an adverse outcome, but in the adequacy of diagnosis, documentation, informed consent, and timely management. A mature clinician understands that failure analysis is a structured diagnostic exercise rather than an emotional response. Effective management requires biological reasoning, technical reassessment, transparent communication, and ethical responsibility.

Diagnosis of failure begins with categorization. Biological failures include recurrent caries, periodontal breakdown, pulpal necrosis, and peri-implantitis. Mechanical failures encompass fracture of restorative materials, loss of retention, screw loosening, and prosthetic component breakage. Functional failures involve occlusal disharmony, temporomandibular discomfort, and phonetic disturbances. Aesthetic failures include shade mismatch, contour discrepancies, and soft tissue asymmetry. Accurate identification of the failure domain prevents inappropriate corrective measures.

Consider a scenario in which a recently placed posterior composite restoration fractures within six months. Superficial interpretation might attribute this solely to material weakness. A structured diagnostic review may reveal that the patient is a nocturnal bruxer with heavy occlusal forces and that cusp coverage was not provided despite thin remaining enamel.

The failure, therefore, reflects biomechanical overload rather than adhesive inadequacy. Revision strategy in such a case requires occlusal risk management, possibly with indirect cusp coverage and protective splint therapy, rather than simple replacement of the same restoration.

Endodontic failure presents another illustrative scenario. A tooth treated for necrotic pulp develops persistent periapical radiolucency after one year. Diagnosis requires assessment of obturation density, missed canals, coronal seal integrity, and presence of vertical root fracture. Cone-beam imaging may reveal an untreated accessory canal. If the cause is identifiable and correctable, nonsurgical retreatment offers a biologically sound revision pathway. However, if fracture or extensive resorption is confirmed, extraction becomes the rational solution. The clinician must communicate clearly that failure does not necessarily imply procedural negligence but may arise from anatomical complexity or microbial persistence. Implant complications demand particularly careful evaluation because patient expectations are often high. Early implant failure may result from inadequate primary stability or systemic risk factors such as uncontrolled diabetes or smoking. Late complications frequently involve peri-implantitis secondary to plaque accumulation or prosthetic overload. Revision may include debridement, regenerative procedures, occlusal adjustment, or in severe cases, implant removal. Importantly, management should be proactive and evidence-based; delay in addressing peri-implant inflammation can convert a manageable complication into irreversible bone loss.

Periodontal surgical failures often reflect incomplete risk control. A regenerative procedure performed in a smoker without cessation counseling may show limited bone fill. In such cases, the revision strategy focuses first on modifying risk factors before repeating surgery. Attempting repeated surgical correction without addressing etiologic contributors risks further attachment loss and patient dissatisfaction.

Aesthetic failures, though biologically benign, may generate disproportionate dissatisfaction. A ceramic crown placed in the anterior region may be technically acceptable but mismatched in translucency. Revision strategy requires shade reassessment, laboratory communication, and realistic discussion of limitations. The clinician must balance the psychological impact of aesthetic concerns with biological preservation. Removing a well-functioning crown solely for minor shade variation requires careful consent and documentation.

Communication forms the cornerstone of medico-legal protection. When complications arise, early disclosure and empathetic explanation reduce adversarial escalation. Patients who perceive transparency and commitment to resolution are less likely to pursue litigation. Conversely, defensive denial or delayed acknowledgment increases mistrust. Documentation should record baseline diagnosis, treatment plan alternatives, consent discussion, procedural notes, postoperative instructions, and follow-up findings. In many medico-legal cases, the absence of documentation—not the complication itself—determines liability.

Consider a case in which a mandibular implant placement results in transient paresthesia. If preoperative imaging documented safe distance from the inferior alveolar nerve and informed consent included nerve injury risk, the occurrence may be classified as a known complication. However, absence of radiographic planning or risk disclosure could reclassify the same outcome as negligent.

Revision strategies should adhere to a hierarchy of conservatism. First, identify and eliminate the etiological factor. Second, evaluate whether conservative correction is feasible. Third, consider more invasive alternatives only if prognosis justifies escalation. Repeating the same procedure without understanding cause perpetuates failure cycles. For example, repeatedly recementing a crown without addressing short axial wall height fails to correct the underlying retention deficiency.

Psychological management of failure is equally important. Patients may interpret failure as betrayal of trust. Professional composure, acknowledgment of concern, and collaborative planning restore therapeutic alliance. Blaming materials, laboratories, or patients erodes credibility. Ethical practice requires ownership of outcome while objectively analyzing causation.

From a systems perspective, complication analysis contributes to clinical quality improvement. Audit of failure patterns—such as recurrent caries around certain margin designs or frequent debonding of specific materials—can refine protocols. Continuous professional development reduces recurrence risk and strengthens standard-of-care adherence.

In conclusion, managing complications and failures is not merely corrective intervention but diagnostic reevaluation, risk modification, transparent communication, and ethical accountability. Dentistry operates within biological uncertainty; therefore, the clinician's responsibility lies not in guaranteeing perfection but in ensuring rational decision-making, informed consent, meticulous documentation, and timely corrective action. A complication managed competently may strengthen professional credibility, whereas one concealed or mismanaged may undermine it irrevocably.

Integrated Table: Managing Complications and Failures in Clinical Dentistry

Type of Failure	Clinical Scenario	Probable Etiology	Diagnostic Approach	Revision Strategy	Medico-Legal Consideration
Restorative (Biological)	Recurrent caries under composite within 1 year	Inadequate isolation, high caries risk, marginal leakage	Clinical exam, bitewing radiograph, caries risk	Remove restoration, caries control protocol, improved isolation, consider	Document initial caries risk, isolation method, and patient

			reassess ment	material change	hygiene instructi ons
Restora tive (Mecha nical)	Fracture d posterio r composi te	Occlusal overload, insufficie nt cusp coverage	Occlusa l analysis , parafun ction assessm ent	Replace with indirect onlay/cro wn, consider occlusal guard	Record occlusal findings and rational e for revised material choice
Endodo ntic Failure	Persiste nt periapic al radioluc ency post-RCT	Missed canal, coronal leakage, fracture	Clinical testing, radiogra phs, CBCT if indicate d	Nonsurgi cal retreatme nt or surgical endodont ics; extract if non-restorabl e	Maintai n docume ntation of preoper ative status, consent, and anatomi cal challeng es
Prostho dontic Failure	Debond ed crown	Short axial wall height, cement failure	Evaluat e preparat ion geometr y, occlusio n	Redesign preparati on, use adhesive cement, or modify prostheti	Docume nt preparat ion paramet ers and cement selectio

				c plan	n rationale
Implant Early Failure	Implant mobility within 3 months	Poor primary stability, systemic risk factors	Clinical mobility test, radiographic evaluation	Remove implant, allow healing, reassess systemic and local factors before reattempt	Document systemic risk disclosure and preoperative imaging
Peri-Implantitis (Late Failure)	Bleeding, bone loss around implant	Plaque accumulation, overload	Probing, radiographic bone assessment	Mechanical debridement, antimicrobial therapy, regenerative approach if feasible	Document maintenance instructions and recall compliance
Periodontal Surgical Failure	Limited regeneration after graft	Smoking, poor plaque control	Risk reassessment, plaque index	Reinforce risk control before considering revision surgery	Record preoperative risk factor counseling

Occlusal/TMD Complication	Persistent jaw pain after occlusal adjustment	Incorrect diagnosis, muscular etiology	Reevaluate TMD classification	Reversible therapy (splint, physiotherapy)	Avoid irreversible adjustments without documented diagnosis
Aesthetic Dissatisfaction	Shade mismatch in anterior crown	Inaccurate shade selection, lab communication gap	Photographic comparison, patient feedback	Remake restoration after revised shade protocol	Preoperative photographs and aesthetic consent critical
Surgical Complication	Post-extraction paresthesia	Nerve proximity, surgical trauma	Neurosensory testing, imaging	Monitor if transient; refer if persistent	Preoperative imaging and nerve injury risk disclosure essential

Patient Communication and Ethical Decisions

Dr. Yashavanth A
Reader, Dept of OMFS
Sri Rajiv Gandhi college of Dental Sciences
Chola nagar, Bangalore 560032

Informed consent, shared decision-making, ethics, and cost-benefit discussions.

Patient communication is not merely a procedural requirement in dentistry; it is a foundational clinical skill that shapes outcomes, trust, compliance, and medico-legal security. Ethical decision-making extends beyond choosing the technically correct treatment. It involves aligning biological possibilities with patient values, financial realities, risk tolerance, and long-term prognosis. Modern dental practice increasingly emphasizes partnership rather than paternalism, shifting from "doctor decides" to structured shared decision-making grounded in transparency and professional integrity.

Informed consent is often misunderstood as a signed document. In reality, it is a communicative process. Ethically and legally, valid consent requires disclosure of diagnosis, nature of proposed treatment, reasonable alternatives, risks and benefits, and the consequences of declining treatment. The clinician must also assess patient understanding and voluntariness. Without comprehension, consent is incomplete. Without discussion of alternatives, it may be considered biased. Without documentation, it becomes indefensible.

Shared decision-making becomes particularly important in cases where multiple acceptable treatment pathways exist, such as endodontic therapy versus extraction and implant placement, direct composite restoration versus indirect ceramic onlay, or nonsurgical periodontal therapy versus surgical intervention. In such scenarios, the dentist's role is to present evidence-based options, clarify prognosis, and contextualize risks, while the patient integrates personal priorities such as aesthetics, cost, time, fear, or systemic health considerations.

Ethical principles guiding dental decisions traditionally include autonomy, beneficence, nonmaleficence, and justice. Autonomy supports a patient's right to accept or refuse treatment, even when refusal may compromise prognosis. Beneficence requires acting in the patient's best interest. Nonmaleficence obligates avoidance of unnecessary harm, including overtreatment. Justice demands fairness in recommendations regardless of socioeconomic status. Ethical tension arises when these principles conflict—for example, when a patient demands an extraction of a restorable tooth for financial reasons. The clinician must balance respect for autonomy with professional responsibility to avoid irreversible harm.

Cost–benefit discussions are often uncomfortable but ethically essential. Financial transparency prevents misunderstanding and reinforces trust. A treatment that is biologically ideal but economically inaccessible is not clinically realistic. Offering phased treatment plans, alternative materials, or staged care may preserve function while accommodating patient constraints. However, presenting lower-cost options must not equate to presenting substandard care. The key lies in explaining trade-offs honestly rather than implicitly steering decisions.

The following integrated table outlines major communication and ethical decision domains in clinical dentistry.

Communication and Ethical Decision Framework:

Decision Domain	Clinical Context	Ethical Principle Involved	Communication Strategy	Risk if Mishandled	Documentation Priority
Informe	Surgica	Autonom	Explain	Allegati	Signed

d Consent	l extraction, implant placement	y, nonmaleficence	procedure, risks (nerve injury, infection), alternatives, and no-treatment outcome	on of undisclosed risk	consent plus narrative note of discussion
Shared Decision-Making	RCT vs extraction + implant	Autonomy, beneficence	Present survival rates, cost, time, long-term maintenance	Perception of bias or overtreatment	Record options discussed and patient preference
Financial Ethics	High-cost full-mouth rehabilitation	Justice	Provide phased options, written estimate	Financial dispute or perceived coercion	Written cost breakdown and payment discussion note
Treatment Refusal	Patient declines periodontal surgery	Autonomy	Clarify consequences of refusal without pressure	Claim of abandonment or neglect	Refusal acknowledgment form

Overtreatment Risk	Replacing intact amalgam for cosmetic reasons	Nonmaleficence	Discuss risks of removal, pulpal trauma	Ethical violation, board complaint	Record patient-driven request
Under-treatment Risk	Delaying caries treatment due to cost	Beneficence	Explain disease progression and interim measures	Disease progression blamed on clinician	Note recommendations and patient decision
Aesthetic Expectations	Veneer case dissatisfaction	Autonomy, beneficence	Use photographs, mock-ups, realistic previews	Unrealistic expectations and dispute	Pre-op images and aesthetic consent
Complex Prognosis	Tooth with guarded periodontal prognosis	Honesty, beneficence	Use percentages and clear timelines	Misunderstood survival expectations	Written prognosis discussion
Second Opinion Request	Patient seeks confirm	Autonomy	Encourage without defensive	Perceived insecurit	Document referral

s	ation		ness	y or conceal ment	
End-of-Life Dental Decisio ns	Medica lly compro mised elderly patient	Nonmale ficence	Focus on comfort, minimal invasiven ess	Overtrea tment of frail patient	Medica l consult ation record

The Psychology of Consent and Comprehension

Research consistently shows that patients retain limited technical detail after consultations. Therefore, effective communication relies on structured clarity rather than dense explanation. Use of diagrams, intraoral photographs, radiographic visuals, and simplified risk percentages enhances comprehension. For example, explaining that "this tooth has an 80–85 percent chance of surviving five years with root canal therapy" is clearer than stating "good prognosis." Similarly, stating "without treatment, infection may spread and cause pain or swelling" is more concrete than saying "possible complications."

The teach-back method—asking the patient to explain in their own words what they understand—helps ensure clarity. This is particularly important before surgical or irreversible procedures.

Managing Ethical Dilemmas in Complex Cases

Consider a patient requesting extraction of a strategically important molar because implant advertising suggests it is "more modern." Ethically, the clinician must explain that preserving natural dentition generally offers biomechanical and proprioceptive advantages. Extracting a restorable tooth for convenience without proper justification may violate nonmaleficence. However, if the patient understands the risks and still prefers extraction after balanced counseling, autonomy prevails—provided documentation reflects the process.

In contrast, consider a patient insisting on aggressive cosmetic treatment despite high caries risk and poor oral hygiene. Proceeding without first stabilizing disease would likely compromise long-term success. Here, beneficence and nonmaleficence override cosmetic desire. Ethical care may require deferring elective treatment until risk factors are controlled.

Cost–Benefit Transparency and Phased Treatment Planning

Cost discussions should occur early and be structured. A useful approach includes three tiers of planning: ideal comprehensive care, alternative conservative care, and interim stabilization. For example, in a partially edentulous patient, options may include implant-supported fixed prosthesis, removable partial denture, or transitional acrylic appliance. Presenting these side by side empowers the patient and demonstrates fairness.

Transparency also reduces allegations of financial motivation. When documentation reflects that less expensive alternatives were discussed, it strengthens ethical defensibility.

Communicating Risk Without Fear

Overemphasizing risk may generate unnecessary anxiety, while underemphasizing risk may appear deceptive. Balanced language is critical. For example, during implant consent, the clinician should disclose risks such as infection, implant failure, or nerve disturbance while emphasizing that complication rates are relatively low when proper case selection is followed. Avoiding technical jargon while maintaining accuracy strengthens trust.

Ethical Documentation

Documentation is both clinical memory and legal safeguard. Notes should include diagnostic findings, options presented, patient questions, expressed concerns, and final decisions. Statements such as "Discussed RCT vs extraction and implant; patient prefers RCT to preserve natural tooth; understands possibility of retreatment" demonstrate transparency.

In aesthetic or elective cases, photographic documentation before and after treatment provides objective reference if disputes arise. For high-risk surgical cases, written acknowledgement of specific complications—such as sinus exposure or paresthesia risk—may be critical.

Cultural Sensitivity and Autonomy

Cultural background may influence decision-making styles. Some patients prefer directive guidance; others want detailed data. Some may defer decisions to family members. Ethical communication respects these preferences while ensuring the individual patient retains final authority.

Communication in Adverse Events

When complications occur, transparent disclosure is ethically mandated. Attempting concealment erodes trust and increases legal exposure. A structured approach includes acknowledging the event, explaining the management plan, offering appropriate remediation, and documenting the discussion. Studies consistently show that honesty reduces litigation risk compared to defensiveness.

Ethical Referrals

Recognizing limits is a professional strength. Referring complex endodontic retreatment, advanced periodontal surgery, or full-arch implant rehabilitation to a specialist reflects commitment to beneficence. Documentation should reflect that referral was offered or recommended.

Decision Tree Framework for Ethical Clinical Communication

Below is a structured conceptual model guiding patient-centered decision-making:

Step	Clinical Action	Communication Focus	Ethical Anchor
1	Establish diagnosis	Use visual aids	Honesty
2	Define urgency	Clarify disease progression	Beneficence

3	Present options	Compare outcomes and costs	Autonomy
4	Discuss risks	Balanced probability explanation	Nonmaleficence
5	Assess understanding	Teach-back method	Respect
6	Confirm decision	Voluntary agreement	Autonomy
7	Document	Detailed narrative entry	Accountability
8	Plan follow-up	Reinforce maintenance	Continuity of care

Practical Example Scenario

A 45-year-old patient presents with a cracked mandibular molar. Options include full-coverage crown, extraction with implant, or extraction with removable prosthesis. The clinician explains crack extent, pulp vitality status, survival probability of crown (approximately 10–15 years if periodontal support remains stable), higher cost but long-term predictability of implant, and lower cost but functional limitations of removable replacement. The patient expresses moderate financial limitation and desire to preserve natural tooth. After discussion, crown placement is selected. Documentation includes risk of future endodontic therapy, possibility of fracture propagation, and patient acknowledgment.

If five years later the tooth fractures vertically and requires extraction, prior documentation of informed risk discussion demonstrates ethical transparency rather than treatment failure.

Digital, AI, and Future-Focused Decision Tools

Dr. Rajesh Patnaik
Senior lecturer
Department of Periodontics
M R Ambedkar Dental College and Hospital,
cline road, bangalore: 560005

Clinical decision support systems, AI diagnostics, and personalized

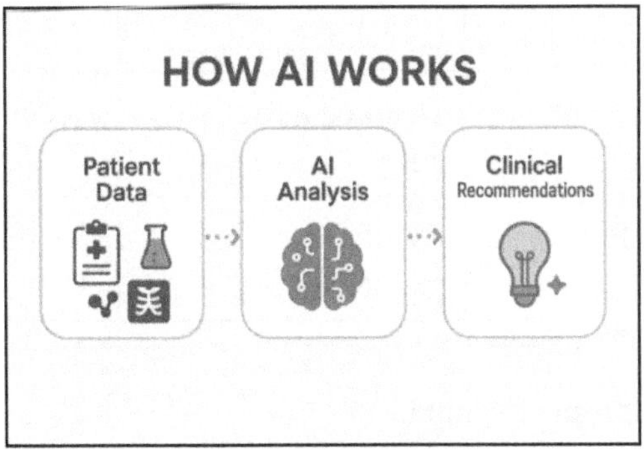

Clinical Decision Support Systems, AI Diagnostics, and Personalized Dentistry

The evolution of dentistry into a digitally integrated healthcare discipline is transforming clinical decision-making from intuition-based judgment supported by static records into data-driven, predictive, and personalized care. Digital imaging, artificial intelligence (AI), machine learning algorithms, and clinical decision support systems (CDSS) are increasingly influencing how diagnoses are made, risks are calculated, and treatment plans are designed. While traditional diagnostic reasoning remains foundational, digital augmentation enhances precision, reduces variability, and supports evidence-based consistency.

Clinical Decision Support Systems are structured digital platforms that analyze patient data and provide evidence-aligned recommendations. These systems integrate radiographs, periodontal charting, caries risk assessment tools, medical histories, and sometimes even genomic information. Rather than replacing the clinician, CDSS functions as an analytical assistant, highlighting potential pathology, suggesting risk levels, and prompting guideline-based interventions. For example, in caries management, AI-enhanced radiographic analysis may identify proximal lesions at earlier stages than the human eye, prompting remineralization strategies rather than operative intervention.

AI diagnostics rely on pattern recognition trained on large datasets. In dental radiology, AI algorithms can detect periapical radiolucencies, marginal bone loss, vertical root fractures, and implant-related bone defects with high sensitivity. However, sensitivity does not equal clinical context. The clinician must interpret findings within biological, symptomatic, and restorative frameworks. AI can detect radiographic bone loss, but it cannot independently determine whether that loss is stable, progressive, or clinically significant without human correlation.

Personalized dentistry represents the convergence of digital risk modeling, behavioral analytics, and sometimes genetic predisposition. Caries risk assessment platforms, for instance, combine salivary flow rate, bacterial load, dietary frequency, fluoride exposure, and previous disease history to generate individualized prevention plans. Similarly, periodontal risk calculators incorporate smoking status, diabetes control, plaque indices, and pocket depths to predict disease progression probability. These tools move dentistry toward preventive precision rather than reactive intervention. Despite these advances, digital systems introduce ethical, legal, and practical considerations. Algorithmic bias, data privacy, over-reliance on automation, and liability allocation must be carefully navigated. AI recommendations should support—not dictate—clinical judgment. Overdependence risks deskilling practitioners, while underutilization forfeits potential benefits.

The following integrated table outlines core categories of digital and AI-driven decision tools in modern dentistry.

Integrated Table: Digital and AI Decision Tools in Dentistry

Tool Category	Clinical Application	Decision Impact	Advantages	Limitations	Ethical Consideration
AI Radiographic Analysis	Caries detection, periapical lesions, bone loss	Early diagnosis, reduced oversight	High sensitivity, consistency	False positives, limited contextual understanding	Must verify findings clinically
Clinical Decision Support Systems (CDSS)	Treatment planning prompts	Guideline-based care standardization	Evidence integration	Over-reliance risk	Clinician remains final decision-maker
Digital Caries Risk Assessment Platforms	Preventive planning	Personalized recall intervals	Data-driven prevention	Requires accurate input data	Transparency in risk explanation
Digital Periodontal Charting with Analytics	Disease progression tracking	Maintenance interval adjustment	Objective monitoring	Software learning curve	Secure storage of patient data
CBCT with AI	Implant plannin	Anatomical	3D visualiz	Radiation	Justification of

Segmentation	g, endodontic assessment	precision	ation	exposure concerns	imaging necessity
Intraoral Scanners + CAD/CAM	Digital impressions, prosthetic fabrication	Improved marginal accuracy	Reduced distortion	Equipment cost	Disclosure of digital workflow
Predictive Implant Stability Algorithms	Primary stability forecasting	Improved case selection	Risk stratification	Limited by dataset scope	Informed consent about predictive uncertainty
Teledentistry Platforms	Remote triage and follow-up	Access expansion	Convenience	Diagnostic limitations	Data confidentiality
Genomic /Salivary Diagnostics	Caries and periodontal susceptibility	Personalized prevention	Precision risk modeling	Emerging evidence base	Patient data protection
AI Occlusal	Bite force	Occlusal adjustme	Quantifiable	Interpretation	Avoid unnece

Analysis Systems	distribution mapping	nt planning	metrics	variability	ssary irreversible treatment

Clinical Integration of AI into Decision-Making

Consider a patient presenting with asymptomatic posterior teeth. AI-assisted radiographic software flags early proximal demineralization. Without AI support, these lesions might be overlooked until cavitation occurs. The clinician confirms findings clinically, correlates with caries risk assessment, and opts for fluoride varnish and dietary counseling rather than operative treatment. Here, AI enhances early prevention rather than promoting overtreatment.

In implant planning, CBCT integrated with digital planning software allows virtual implant placement considering bone density, sinus proximity, and prosthetic alignment. AI-driven segmentation highlights inferior alveolar nerve trajectory, reducing surgical risk. However, the clinician must still evaluate systemic health, smoking status, occlusal loading, and maintenance compliance before proceeding.

In endodontics, AI may detect subtle periapical pathology invisible to the naked eye. Yet clinical correlation with pulp testing and symptomatology determines treatment necessity. An isolated radiographic finding without symptoms may warrant monitoring rather than intervention.

Decision Tree Framework for AI-Supported Clinical Care

Step	Clinical Action	Digital Integration	Safeguard
1	Gather diagnostic data	Digital radiographs,	Ensure data quality

		scans	
2	AI analysis	Algorithmic detection	Cross-check manually
3	Clinical correlation	Symptoms + exam	Avoid automation bias
4	Risk modelling	Predictive analytics	Explain uncertainty
5	Treatment planning	Digital simulation	Maintain patient-centered discussion
6	Consent	Discuss digital tools used	Transparency
7	Implementation	Guided workflow	Document software support
8	Follow-up analytics	Progress tracking	Human interpretation required

Automation Bias and Clinical Responsibility

Automation bias occurs when clinicians over-trust AI outputs, even when contradictory evidence exists. For example, if AI fails to detect a small periapical lesion that the clinician observes clinically, deferring to AI could delay diagnosis. Conversely, treating every AI-flagged anomaly without contextual evaluation may lead to overtreatment. Therefore, digital systems should function as adjunctive verification tools.

Professional accountability remains with the dentist, not the software developer. If an AI recommendation contributes to an adverse outcome, responsibility typically resides with the clinician who accepted the recommendation. This underscores the importance of maintaining independent diagnostic reasoning.

Personalized Preventive Dentistry

Future-focused dentistry increasingly emphasizes predictive modeling. Salivary biomarkers may identify inflammatory mediators linked to periodontal susceptibility. Genetic profiling may reveal variations influencing enamel strength or immune response. Behavioral analytics integrated with digital toothbrush tracking could customize recall intervals and preventive reinforcement strategies.

For example, a patient with controlled diabetes, moderate plaque levels, and genetic markers suggesting higher inflammatory response may benefit from three-month periodontal maintenance rather than the traditional six-month interval. Personalized recall systems reduce both undertreatment and unnecessary visits.

Economic and Practice Implications

Digital integration requires financial investment in scanners, CBCT units, software subscriptions, and training. However, improved diagnostic accuracy, patient engagement through visual simulation, and streamlined workflows may enhance efficiency and case acceptance. Patients increasingly perceive digitally equipped practices as modern and trustworthy.

Transparency regarding digital tools strengthens patient confidence. Explaining that AI-assisted radiograph analysis supports diagnosis reinforces thoroughness rather than automation dependence.

Data Privacy and Ethical Safeguards

With increased digital integration comes responsibility for data security. Patient imaging, biometric information, and health analytics must be stored in secure, encrypted systems compliant with healthcare privacy regulations. Unauthorized data exposure can result in significant legal and reputational harm.

Informed consent should include disclosure when advanced digital analytics or AI-assisted diagnostics are used, particularly when cloud-based platforms process patient data.

The Future Landscape

Emerging technologies include real-time caries detection via optical coherence tomography, robotic-assisted implant placement, augmented reality surgical guides, and AI-driven full-mouth rehabilitation simulation. Digital twins—virtual replicas of patient dentition—may allow predictive modeling of occlusal wear and restorative longevity.

Integration of systemic health records with dental analytics may further refine risk modeling. For example, cardiovascular data, glycemic control indices, and inflammatory markers could influence periodontal maintenance intervals.

Balanced Perspective

Despite enthusiasm for innovation, technology cannot replace clinical empathy, tactile assessment, or ethical judgment. Digital tools enhance pattern recognition and data processing but cannot evaluate patient anxiety, financial hardship, or nuanced aesthetic expectations. The future of dentistry lies not in automation but in augmentation—where digital precision complements human reasoning.

Conclusion

Digital, AI, and future-focused decision tools are reshaping dentistry toward predictive, personalized, and minimally invasive care. Clinical Decision Support Systems and AI diagnostics enhance accuracy and consistency, while personalized analytics improve preventive strategies. However, these technologies demand careful ethical oversight, continued professional judgment, and transparent patient communication. The clinician remains the central decision-maker, integrating digital intelligence with biological understanding and human-centered care.

Reference

1. Stefanac SJ, Nesbit SP. *Diagnosis and Treatment Planning in Dentistry.* Foundational text addressing systematic diagnostic frameworks and structured treatment sequencing in clinical dentistry.
2. Jeske AH (Ed.). *Mosby's Dental Drug Reference.* Comprehensive pharmacologic guide for dental therapeutics, drug interactions, and prescription protocols.
3. Anusavice KJ, Shen C, Rawls HR. *Phillips' Science of Dental Materials.* Authoritative reference on the physical, mechanical, and biological properties of dental materials.
4. Aschheim KW, Dale BG. *Esthetic Dentistry: A Clinical Approach to Techniques and Materials.* Clinical protocols for cosmetic restorative procedures and smile design principles.
5. Ash MM Jr., Nelson SJ. *Wheeler's Dental Anatomy, Physiology, and Occlusion.* Classic resource on tooth morphology, occlusal relationships, and functional dynamics.
6. Avery JK, Chiego DJ. *Essentials of Oral Histology and Embryology: A Clinical Approach.* Microscopic anatomy and developmental biology correlated with clinical practice.
7. Bagg J, MacFarlane TW, Poxton IR, Smith AJ. *Essentials of Microbiology for Dental Students.* Oral microbiology principles relevant to infection and disease progression.
8. McCabe JF, Walls AWG. *Dental Materials: Properties and Manipulation.* Practical overview of restorative materials and clinical handling techniques.
9. Rosenstiel SF, Land MF, Fujimoto J. *Contemporary Fixed Prosthodontics.* Evidence-based principles for crowns, bridges, and fixed prosthetic restorations.
10. Carr AB, Brown DT. *McCracken's Removable Partial Prosthodontics.* Comprehensive guide to removable prosthesis

design and biomechanics.

11. Hargreaves KM, Berman LH (Eds.). *Cohen's Pathways of the Pulp.* Definitive text on endodontic biology, diagnosis, and treatment.

12. Ten Cate AR. *Orban's Oral Histology and Embryology.* Detailed exploration of oral tissues and developmental processes.

13. Balaji SM. *Textbook of Oral and Maxillofacial Surgery.* Surgical principles and procedures in maxillofacial practice.

14. Fonseca RJ (Ed.). *Contemporary Oral and Maxillofacial Surgery.* Modern surgical techniques and evidence-based management.

15. Peterson LJ et al. *Peterson's Principles of Oral and Maxillofacial Surgery.* Foundational surgical reference text.

16. Cawson RA, Odell EW. *Cawson's Essentials of Oral Pathology and Oral Medicine.* Core pathology and oral medicine resource.

17. Greenberg MS, Glick M, Ship JA. *Burket's Oral Medicine.* Diagnosis and management of medically complex dental patients.

18. Newman MG, Takei HH, Klokkevold PR, Carranza FA. *Carranza's Clinical Periodontology.* Gold-standard reference for periodontal diagnosis and therapy.

19. Gehrig JS, Willmann DE. *Foundations of Periodontics for the Dental Hygienist.* Periodontal instrumentation and maintenance strategies.

20. Carranza FA. *Glickman's Clinical Periodontology.* Historical cornerstone in periodontal science and therapy.

21. Summitt JB, Hilton TJ, Robbins JW, Schwartz RS. *Fundamentals of Operative Dentistry: A Contemporary Approach.* Conservative restorative principles.

22. Ritter AV et al. *Sturdevant's Art and Science of Operative Dentistry.* Advanced operative techniques and restorative philosophy.

23. Grossman LI, Oliet S, Del Rio CE. *Grossman's Endodontic Practice.* Classical reference in endodontic therapy.

24. White SC, Pharoah MJ. *Oral Radiology: Principles and Interpretation.* Diagnostic imaging principles and radiographic interpretation.

25. Iannucci JM, Howerton LJ. *Dental Radiography: Principles and Techniques.* Radiographic positioning and safety protocols.

26. Hansen JT. *Netter's Clinical Anatomy.* Visual atlas of head and neck anatomy for clinical application.

27. Proffit WR, Fields HW, Larson BE, Sarver DM. *Contemporary Orthodontics.* Comprehensive orthodontic diagnosis and biomechanics.

28. Malamed SF. *Handbook of Local Anesthesia.* Authoritative reference on dental anesthesia techniques and complications.

29. Shafer WG, Hine MK, Levy BM. *Shafer's Textbook of Oral Pathology.* Fundamental oral pathology text.

30. Lindhe J, Lang NP, Berglundh T (Eds.). *Clinical Periodontology and Implant Dentistry.* Integration of periodontal and implant sciences.

31. Fejerskov O, Nyvad B, Kidd E (Eds.). *Caries: The Disease and Its Clinical Management.* Biological understanding of dental caries and prevention strategies.

32. Monheim LM. *Local Anesthesia and Pain Control in Dental Practice.* Clinical anesthesia techniques.

33. Samaranayake LP. *Essential Microbiology for Dentistry.* Oral microbial ecology and pathogenesis.

34. Tripathi KD. *Essentials of Medical Pharmacology.* Foundational pharmacology relevant to dental prescribing.

35. Robbins SL, Cotran RS. *Robbins and Cotran Pathologic Basis of Disease.* Systemic pathology correlation.

36. Brown WH, Herbranson EJ. *Dental Anatomy and Occlusion.* Morphology and occlusal concepts.

37. Little JW, Falace DA, Miller CS, Rhodus NL. *Dental Management of the Medically Compromised Patient.* Risk assessment in medically complex patients.

38. Soben Peter. *Textbook of Preventive and Community Dentistry.* Public oral health principles.

39. Rang HP et al. *Rang and Dale's Pharmacology.* Systemic pharmacologic principles.

40. Fonseca RJ. *Oral and Maxillofacial Surgery (3-volume set).* Comprehensive surgical resource.
41. Okeson JP. *Management of Temporomandibular Disorders and Occlusion.* Diagnostic and therapeutic approach to TMD.
42. Dawson PE. *Functional Occlusion: From TMJ to Smile Design.* Occlusal philosophy and clinical integration.
43. Misch CE. *Dental Implant Prosthetics.* Biomechanics and implant-supported restoration planning.
44. Nevins M, Mellonig JT. *Periodontal and Implant Therapy.* Regenerative and surgical approaches.
45. Kumar V, Abbas AK, Aster JC. *Robbins Basic Pathology.* Medical pathology foundation.
46. Mount GJ, Hume WR. *Preservation and Restoration of Tooth Structure.* Minimally invasive restorative philosophy.
47. Heymann HO, Swift EJ, Ritter AV. *Sturdevant's Art and Science of Operative Dentistry.* Contemporary operative reference.
48. Proffit WR. *Orthodontic Diagnosis and Treatment Planning.* Clinical orthodontic strategies.
49. Fonseca RJ, Barber HD. *Oral and Maxillofacial Trauma.* Trauma management protocols.
50. Feinberg SE, Larson BE. *Orthognathic Surgery: Principles and Practice.* Surgical orthodontic correction guidelines.
51. Ingle JI, Bakland LK, Baumgartner JC. *Ingle's Endodontics.* Comprehensive reference on endodontic biology, instrumentation, obturation, and retreatment strategies.
52. Peterson LJ, Ellis E, Hupp JR, Tucker MR. *Contemporary Oral and Maxillofacial Surgery.* Surgical procedures, principles of exodontia, and management of pathologic lesions.
53. Misch CE. *Contemporary Implant Dentistry.* Evidence-based implant planning, biomechanics, and prosthetic considerations.
54. Lindhe J, Karring T, Lang NP. *Clinical Periodontology and Implant*

Dentistry. Integration of periodontal science with implant therapy and regenerative procedures.

55. Featherstone JDB, Kidd EAM, Nyvad B. *Dental Caries: The Disease and Its Clinical Management.* Scientific understanding of caries etiology and preventive strategies.

56. Okeson JP. *Management of Temporomandibular Disorders and Occlusion.* Diagnostic classification and therapeutic approaches to TMD.

57. Dawson PE. *Functional Occlusion: From TMJ to Smile Design.* Comprehensive occlusal philosophy linking function and esthetics.

58. Heymann HO, Swift EJ, Ritter AV. *Sturdevant's Art and Science of Operative Dentistry.* Advanced operative techniques and biomimetic restorative principles.

59. Summitt JB, Hilton TJ, Robbins JW, Schwartz RS. *Fundamentals of Operative Dentistry.* Conservative restorative protocols emphasizing minimal intervention.

60. Proffit WR, Fields HW, Sarver DM. *Contemporary Orthodontics.* Orthodontic biomechanics, growth modification, and treatment planning.

61. Graber LW, Vanarsdall RL, Vig KWL. *Orthodontics: Current Principles and Techniques.* Clinical orthodontic mechanics and interdisciplinary care.

62. Shafer WG, Hine MK, Levy BM. *Textbook of Oral Pathology.* Foundational reference in oral disease pathology and clinical correlations.

63. Regezi JA, Sciubba JJ, Jordan RCK. *Oral Pathology: Clinical Pathologic Correlations.* Diagnostic integration of clinical and microscopic findings.

64. Greenberg MS, Glick M, Ship JA. *Burket's Oral Medicine.* Diagnosis and management of systemic conditions affecting oral health.

65. White SC, Pharoah MJ. *Oral Radiology: Principles and Interpretation.* Advanced diagnostic imaging techniques and radiographic interpretation.

66. Iannucci JM, Howerton LJ. *Dental Radiography: Principles and Techniques.* Practical radiographic positioning and radiation safety.

67. Malamed SF. *Medical Emergencies in the Dental Office.* Emergency preparedness and management protocols.

68. Little JW, Falace DA, Miller CS, Rhodus NL. *Dental Management of the Medically Compromised Patient.* Clinical adaptations for systemic disease.

69. Carr AB, Brown DT. *McCracken's Removable Partial Prosthodontics.* Biomechanics and clinical procedures for removable prostheses.

70. Rosenstiel SF, Land MF, Fujimoto J. *Contemporary Fixed Prosthodontics.* Tooth preparation design and fixed prosthesis fabrication.

71. Zarb GA, Bolender CL, Eckert SE. *Prosthodontic Treatment for Edentulous Patients.* Complete denture prosthodontics and implant-supported overdentures.

72. Shillingburg HT, Hobo S, Whitsett LD, Jacobi R, Brackett SE. *Fundamentals of Fixed Prosthodontics.* Preparation geometry and prosthetic biomechanics.

73. Neville BW, Damm DD, Allen CM, Chi AC. *Oral and Maxillofacial Pathology.* Comprehensive pathology reference.

74. Fonseca RJ. *Oral and Maxillofacial Surgery.* Multi-volume surgical reference covering trauma, pathology, and reconstructive procedures.

75. Peterson LJ. *Peterson's Principles of Oral and Maxillofacial Surgery.* Foundational surgical principles and techniques.

76. Misch CE. *Dental Implant Prosthetics.* Prosthetic planning and restorative considerations for implants.

77. Buser D, Belser UC, Wismeijer D. *ITI Treatment Guide.* Evidence-based implant placement and restorative protocols.

78. Fejerskov O, Kidd E. *Dental Caries: The Disease and Its Clinical Management.* Biological basis of caries and preventive dentistry.

79. Mount GJ, Hume WR. *Preservation and Restoration of Tooth Structure.* Minimal intervention dentistry philosophy.

80. McCabe JF, Walls AWG. *Applied Dental Materials.* Clinical application of dental material science.

81. Anusavice KJ. *Phillips' Science of Dental Materials.* Biomaterial properties and clinical implications.

82. Samaranayake LP. *Essential Microbiology for Dentistry.* Oral microbial ecology and infection control.

83. Tripathi KD. *Essentials of Medical Pharmacology.* Drug actions and systemic considerations relevant to dentistry.

84. Rang HP, Dale MM, Ritter JM, Flower RJ. *Rang and Dale's Pharmacology.* Mechanisms of drug action applicable to dental prescribing.

85. Soben Peter. *Textbook of Preventive and Community Dentistry.* Epidemiology and public health strategies in dentistry.

86. Darby ML, Walsh MM. *Dental Hygiene: Theory and Practice.* Preventive care and periodontal instrumentation.

87. Gehrig JS, Willmann DE. *Foundations of Periodontics for the Dental Hygienist.* Clinical periodontal therapy protocols.

88. Okeson JP. *Bell's Oral and Facial Pain.* Differential diagnosis of orofacial pain disorders.

89. Dawson PE. *Evaluation, Diagnosis, and Treatment of Occlusal Problems.* Comprehensive occlusal therapy guide.

90. Kumar V, Abbas AK, Aster JC. *Robbins Basic Pathology.* Systemic pathology integration with oral disease.

91. Robbins SL, Cotran RS. *Pathologic Basis of Disease.* Advanced systemic pathology reference.

92. Hupp JR, Ellis E, Tucker MR. *Contemporary Oral and Maxillofacial Surgery.* Clinical surgical management.

93. Fonseca RJ, Barber HD. *Oral and Maxillofacial Trauma.* Trauma assessment and surgical repair.

94. Graber TM, Vanarsdall RL. *Orthodontics: Principles and*

Techniques. Growth, development, and orthodontic therapy.

95. Pinkham JR, Casamassimo PS, Fields HW, McTigue DJ, Nowak AJ. *Pediatric Dentistry: Infancy Through Adolescence.* Comprehensive pediatric dental care.

96. Dean JA. *McDonald and Avery's Dentistry for the Child and Adolescent.* Pediatric restorative and preventive dentistry.

97. Featherstone JDB. *Minimal Intervention Dentistry.* Caries risk management and preventive models.

98. Misch CE. *Contemporary Implant Dentistry.* Surgical and prosthetic implant science integration.

99. Nevins M, Mellonig JT. *Periodontal and Implant Therapy.* Regenerative surgical protocols.

100. Sackett DL, Straus SE, Richardson WS, Rosenberg W, Haynes RB. *Evidence-Based Medicine: How to Practice and Teach EBM.* Foundational principles of evidence-based clinical decision-making applicable to dentistry.

9 788199 862548

Printed at Repro India Ltd.